Maya Pines

The
Brain-Changers

Scientists and the new mind-control

Allen Lane

Copyright © Maya Pines, 1973

First published in the United States of America by
Harcourt, Brace, Jovanovich Inc., New York, 1973

Published in Great Britain in 1974

Allen Lane, a Division of Penguin Books Ltd
17 Grosvenor Gardens, London SW1

ISBN 0 7139 0736 3

Printed in Great Britain by
Clarke, Doble & Brendon Ltd, Plymouth

Contents

Acknowledgements

Many brain scientists in America helped me through the maze of current research. They gave generously of their time, explained what they were doing and why, referred me to other researchers, suggested books and papers to read, took the trouble to correct my errors and answered countless questions. Their enthusiasm for their work was contagious.

While none of them can be held responsible for the final product, I am particularly indebted to: Floyd E. Bloom, St Elizabeth's Hospital; Joseph E. Bogen, Ross-Loos Medical Group, Los Angeles; Karl Frank, National Institute of Neurological Diseases and Stroke; Daniel X. Freedman, University of Chicago; Michael S. Gazzaniga, State University of New York, Stony Brook; Elmer and Alyce Green, The Menninger Foundation; Stanislav Grof, Maryland Psychiatric Research Center; Murray E. Jarvik, U C L A; Joe Kamiya, Langley-Porter Neuropsychiatric Institute; Eric R. Kandel, New York University Medical Center; David Krech, University of California, Berkeley; Paul D. MacLean, National Institute of Mental Health; James L. McGaugh, University of California, Irvine; Neal E. Miller, Rockefeller University; Vernon B. Mountcastle, Johns Hopkins University; Ronald E. Myers, National Institute of Neurological Diseases and Stroke; James Olds, California Institute of Technology; Karl H. Pribram, Stanford University; William B. Scoville, Hartford Hospital; Solomon H. Snyder, Johns Hopkins University; and Roger W. Sperry, California Institute of Technology.

7

Acknowledgements

At the National Research Council, Louise Marshall of the Committee on Brain Sciences made many useful suggestions. My editor, Edwin Barber, gave me the impetus for this book. I greatly appreciate his encouragement. And at all times – particularly in moments of crisis – I could count on support from my husband. To all of them, my deepest thanks.

1 A new power over the brain

The most exciting and mysterious part of the universe is not some primitive jungle or the ocean's floor or even a distant planet. It is the magical three-and-a-half pounds of pinkish-grey jelly we carry around inside our skulls – the human brain. This mechanism, the source of all our thoughts and actions, is at the centre of a scientific explosion. Biologists, chemists, psychologists, surgeons, even engineers are converging on it from every point on the scientific spectrum, and what these brain researchers may tell us about its workings will have a profound effect on the future of human life. We will have the power to use our brains more effectively, to control our own brain waves, to improve our memories, to shape babies' brains and to sharpen or suppress various emotions – in ourselves and in others. One can only guess what this power may mean in the future, or how it might be used, but now the major directions of research are clear. This book is a report on that research.

It is all extremely new. The brain itself has been studied for less than a century. Encased in its thick armour of skull, this convoluted mass defied analysis. For thousands of years, few tried, and those who did attempt to explore it sometimes took one look and gave up in despair. Aristotle, the 'father of psychology', taught that the brain was merely a cooling mechanism for the blood, while all the real thinking went on in the heart. Even after Galen corrected this error, there were no adequate tools with which to investigate the brain. When the invention of the microscope and the discovery of electricity at last made it possible for research to begin, generations of Western scientists refrained from violating the human brain, out of respect for it as the seat of man's immortal soul.

Even today, despite broad progress, researchers remain totally ignorant about how the brain performs its basic job: how it transforms 10 watts of electricity and some chemicals into all our thoughts, feelings, dreams, memories – our awareness of being ourselves. It is beyond understanding. But despite their ignorance, scientists have identified several sensitive triggers or control-points in the brain, largely through trial and error, and in the past twenty years they have made astonishing practical progress in controlling various brain functions. They are now approaching the point, for the first time, where they will know how to change not only our moods, but our abilities and to some extent our behaviour.

Today we are turning inwards. Through drugs, meditation, alpha training and other means more people than ever before are trying to change their mental functions. We consume more narcotics, tranquillizers, stimulants and sleeping pills than all the preceding generations combined. But much of this activity is haphazard or pointless, if not downright harmful, and through it all we have only the vaguest notions of how such invasions really affect our brains.

To find out what has been learned about these and other kinds of brain manipulations, I spent two years visiting research laboratories in various parts of the United States, reading hundreds of reports and interviewing some of the scientists who are doing the most exciting work on the brain. For a journalist, it was a mind-boggling whirl. The brain is now being investigated from every imaginable point of view. It has attracted scientists from the widest variety of backgrounds. Some study behaviour, others study particles under a microscope. Some see emotions or bright colours where others see only cells. Some spend their lives next to rows of fetid caged rats, or experimenting with screeching monkeys. Others try to put dying people in a trance. From many different disciplines, each contributes his special vocabulary and jargon. Sometimes they have trouble communicating with each other. Often they disagree – at times quite violently – and sometimes they even disagree with what they themselves have said only a few years before.

Since I could not begin to do justice to a field so vast, so complicated, so difficult, and in which everything was moving so rapidly, I decided to pick a few areas that seemed particularly interesting or significant and report only on those, going whenever possible to the original sources – the living, breathing and usually controversial pioneers themselves.

Among the researchers who studied the brain as a whole, I was struck by the team which first came up with evidence that the brain changes with experience. Drs David Krech, Mark Rosenzweig, Edward Bennett and Marian Diamond of the University of California at Berkeley discovered that when rats are given many challenging toys to play with and problems to solve their brains actually become heavier, thicker and richer. Probably the human brain changes in similar ways, and eventually we may learn what kind of experience produces the most desirable changes.

Another fascinating line of research involves the different talents of our left and right hemispheres – the two equal halves of our brains – which, in most people, perform unequally. Dr Roger Sperry, of the California Institute of Technology, and his associates have begun to sort out these special talents. Some of us are dominated by our left, and others by our right hemispheres. These two entirely different orientations can now to some extent be measured, and perhaps changed.

With the help of computers to unscramble the electrical language of our brains, other scientists are studying the swift changes in our states of consciousness – the Zen-like calm associated with our slower brain waves, the furious activity of our dreams – and how we can learn to produce different kinds of brain rhythms at will.

Probably the largest group of all is trying to solve the mystery

11

of how we learn and how we remember. Here again there are those who investigate the phenomenon as a whole – the broken memory of a forty-seven-year-old man after a brain operation, for instance, or the behaviour of experimental animals whose memory of what they have just learned can be either sharpened or wiped out. But many scientists believe that the key to memory lies somewhere in the mechanism of individual nerve cells. To reach it, one must go back to ever smaller components of the brain.

In the 1950s several technological advances combined to give scientists a better understanding of how messages flow from nerve cell to nerve cell, and how to interfere with them. The human brain has roughly ten thousand million nerve cells, or neurons. Each has a grey cell body from which a relatively long white fibre (the axon) protrudes at one end to make contact with other cells, while a profusion of branch-like fibres (dendrites) at the other end receives perhaps thousands of similar contacts from other axons. Thanks to the electron microscope, it became clear that the fibres of two separate neurons never actually touch: there is always an ultrafine gap at their junction, or synapse. When a neuron fires, an electrical impulse travels down the axon. The impulse releases a chemical transmitter that floats across the tiny gap between the cells, producing an electrical reaction on the other side. If this reaction is strong enough, it causes the next cell to fire, and the process starts all over again.

By stimulating nerve cells with a very mild electric current researchers can reproduce natural nerve impulses. In certain parts of the brain this may produce exactly the same effect – the movement of a hand, for instance – as if the person had actually willed it, or a 'real' sensation. But until synapses were better understood it was not clear why similar results could be produced chemically. In recent years, scientists have learned a great deal about some of the brain's neurotransmitters, though many more remain unknown. They are discovering that depressions or elations can sometimes be traced to the sluggish-

12

ness or speed with which nerve cells release certain transmitters. They are finding out that many mood-changing drugs act by mimicking these transmitters. At the same time, they are beginning to decipher which chemicals are involved in the learning process, and what roles the various chemicals play. The search for the key to learning has drawn some of the world's most enterprising scientists. In its present frenzy it reminds researchers of the race to split the atom or to crack the genetic code.

The part of the brain that has aroused most scientific curiosity so far is the cerebral cortex – the wrinkled sheet of grey matter on the surface of the brain. The cortex forms the outer layer of the two bulging hemispheres that dominate man's brain and that are the most recent products of evolution. In the frog these can barely be distinguished from other bumps on the central brain stem. In the rat they are quite clear. In the cat they appear swollen. They continue to expand as one goes up the evolutionary ladder until, in man, they take up five sixths of the total brain mass. They balloon forward, sideways and backwards, covering and hiding nearly all the old brain below. The cortex looks as if it had been stuffed, folded and then pushed in again to gain more space in the skull; in fact, this may well be what happened, since its convolutions triple its surface area. Not only is this the most accessible brain area; it is also the most distinctly human. Most of our thinking, planning, language, imagination, creativity and capacity for abstraction comes from this convoluted sheet.

War is often the unwitting partner of research. Earlier researchers learned a great deal about the cerebral cortex from the behaviour of soldiers with head injuries and patients with brain tumours and other abnormalities. In addition, they used every possible means to investigate the brains of animals: they cut them, cooled them, burned out certain sections and scooped out others, stimulated them with electric current, extracted fluids, injected chemicals, crosshatched them, spread cream inside them or filled them with a variety of foreign objects, just to see what would happen.

By the end of the Second World War brain scientists could tell very precisely what part of the cortex should be stimulated to produce an action of the arm or leg. They also knew where in his cortex a man would feel the sensation of a squeeze on his hand. But they had precious little idea of what went on in the brain between such inputs and outputs.

For this they needed more sophisticated tools: thinner electrodes, which became available in the 1950s, new chemical staining techniques, micro-miniaturized equipment of all kinds, and especially computers to keep track of what was happening. Soon they were able to spy on the activity of individual cells in a living brain. Drilling a hole through an animal's skull, they sank exceedingly fine, glass-tipped micro-electrodes into its brain to record electrical changes within specific cells. These changes could then be related to other events in the animal's brain, some of which excited the cell, while others inhibited it from firing. Through such work they learned, for instance, that it takes about 100 milliseconds for the orders from a single motor neuron in a monkey's cortex to be translated into finger action.

They have also shown that specific cells in the cortex of cats and monkeys preprocess information in incredibly specific ways. One cell involved in vision might fire only in response to a bright line at a particular location and slope, while another responds only to a line at a slightly different location and slope. The cells hold a sophisticated alphabet for lines, corners, direction of movement, colour contrast and so on.

At least three quarters of the human cortex has nothing to do with such obvious functions as vision, hearing, touch or muscle movements, however. Much of it is taken up with mysterious activities generally lumped together under the name 'associations'. These may be the key to the subtlety of the human brain, for we have many more such associative areas than do other primates.

Just behind our forehead, for instance, our frontal lobes appear to be deeply involved in planning, in the formation of

14

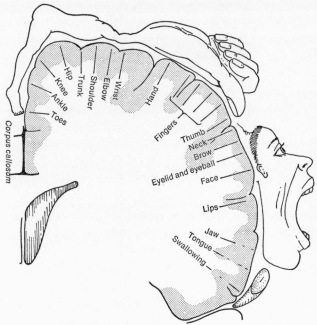

Motor Homunculus of Man
The motor area in the right hemisphere, shown here, controls
actions of the left side of the body. Fingers and mouth take up
more space; they require far more precise control than larger areas
of the body, such as the legs and trunk. After Penfield and Rasmus-
sen. Reprinted by permission of Lea & Febiger from *Functional
Neuroanatomy* by N. B. Everett, 6th edition, 1971.

intentions and programmes, and this the brain scientists are only
beginning to investigate. It is one of the most exciting areas of
brain research, for it touches so vitally on the difference between one's self and others – between our will and acts that are
forced upon us. At the Massachusetts Institute of Technology
researchers have found specific cells in a monkey's frontal cortex
that fire not before a specific eye movement, but during or just
after it, much too soon to be bringing feedback from the eye
muscles. The scientists believe they have found part of the
mechanism of intention. These cells apparently tell the monkey

15

The brain-changers

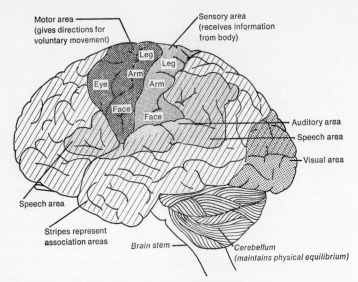

Motor area
(gives directions for
voluntary movement)

Sensory area
(receives information
from body)

Leg

Leg

Arm

Eye

Arm

Face

Face

Auditory area

Speech area

Visual area

Speech area

Stripes represent
association areas

Brain stem

*Cerebellum
(maintains physical equilibrium)*

The Cerebral Cortex (External view of left hemisphere)

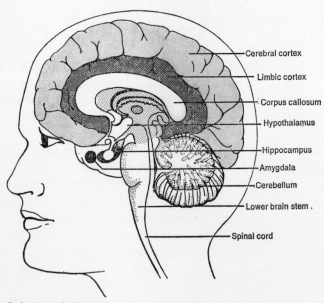

Cerebral cortex

Limbic cortex

Corpus callosum

Hypothalamus

Hippocampus

Amygdala

Cerebellum

Lower brain stem .

Spinal cord

Medial View of the Brain

how it is doing with its plans – where its eyes are moving and what phase of its programme is now in effect. Other MIT scientists have found that unless people or animals can exercise intentional control over their acts, they cannot learn new motor skills.

If the cortex represents our ego, the closest thing to our id is probably the hypothalamus, a small bundle of cells centrally located deep in the brain, near the top of the brain stem. This controls anger, joy, hunger, sex, fear and other drives. The most sensational development in all brain research was probably the discovery of pain and pleasure 'centres' – really circuits – in or near the hypothalami of animals. Stimulation there could be used to reward or punish any kind of behaviour, even from a distance. The two circuits are still very poorly understood, however – they have the unfortunate tendency to become intertwined with each other or mixed up with others, so that the 'pleasure' involved may turn out to be more like a compulsion. José Delgado, of Yale University, one of the scientists who showed that brain pain could make animals learn, and James Olds of the California Institute of Technology, who discovered the pleasure centre, hold diametrically opposed views on what their findings might mean for mankind.

All the older parts of our brain are now being studied with new attention. They all seem involved in our 'gut' reactions, in the primitive emotions that are normally modulated by the cortex. They contain many ancestral memories.

We still have brain structures in our heads much like those of the horse and the crocodile, according to Paul MacLean, a neurophysiologist at the National Institute of Mental Health. Our old reptilian brain, which goes back more than 200 million years in evolution, still directs our mechanisms of courting, mating, finding home sites and selecting leaders. It is responsible for many of our rituals. 'I have a route by which I come to work which is pretty reptilian,' said Dr MacLean. 'I just favour that way, because it seems more comfortable.' The gift some people have for communicating with animals – calming an excited dog, for instance – can also be traced to their reptilian brain. So can the mechanism for personal appeal: Eisenhower's magnetism may have been largely reptilian.

On top of this oldest reptilian brain, which is mostly in the brain stem, the lower mammals built a sort of 'thinking-cap', a primitive cortex that forms a border around the brain stem and is called the limbic system. We still have that, too. 'I can recognize some of my co-workers all the way down the hall, where I can barely see them, by the angle at which they move.' Dr Mac-Lean says. 'It's not my new cortex – my new cortex alone could never recognize them. It's limbic intuitiveness.' The limbic system remains fundamentally the same in all mammals. It continues to do our smelling and tasting, feels what goes on inside our bodies, is involved in memory and plays a key role in our emotions.

What with all these ancient creatures within, and the enormous new cortex that envelops them, how does the human brain decide anything? A generation ago, when the closest equivalent to the brain seemed to be a telephone system, scientists visualized a busy central switchboard with an operator who made all the decisions. This comparison has fallen out of favour. The brain is neither as passive as a switchboard nor so clearly mechanical. Today's scientists prefer to compare the brain to a general-purpose computer with several different elements and memory banks and some built-in (inborn) programmes.

Animals operate largely on built-in programmes. In some ways we do, too – for example, the entire chain of behaviour in the sex act is pre-programmed in our brains. But in addition, we must learn a profusion of new programmes in early childhood or later, and they are the basis of our culture. Our decisions depend very strongly on this cultural conditioning.

People have allowed themselves to be burned at the stake and have murdered other human beings for purely ideological reasons. We are governed by a whole world of abstractions that never affect other animals. Our large cortex produces a complex interplay of associations, memories and learned programmes.

Our forebrain, with its planning areas, allows us to see the possible consequences of our acts. What we will do in any circumstance is never simply the result of an electrical stimulus or a drop of chemical.

This is why some researchers see definite limits to what can be learned from the brains of animals. Those who deal with the smallest units of the brain need not worry about this: a nerve impulse is a nerve impulse. Neurons, transmitters, blood and cerebrospinal fluid are pretty much alike in rat and man. But for those who try to understand learning, or the brain mechanisms which lead to violence, the differences between the brains of animals and men are far more significant. There are major differences in organization, complexity and size, all leading to man's capacity for abstract thought, which is related to language.

According to the MIT linguist Noam Chomsky, man, and only man, is born with a special competence for language. In all cultures of the world, children learn to speak at approximately the same age, as if this were built into their genes. All languages have the same 'deep structures', he has argued, and all children re-invent the rules of grammar for themselves. When a child says 'throwed' instead of 'threw', this shows that he worked out how to make a past tense and applied this rule in an original way to form a word he had never heard before. No animal's brain has the ability to do such a thing.

People whose religious convictions lead them to believe that there is an abrupt discontinuity between men and other creatures find Chomsky's point of view congenial. Those who see man as just another form of life argue that all learning, including language, results from orderly sequences of stimuli, responses and rewards, no different in men from animals.

Until recently, Chomsky's view was supported by the fact that all efforts to teach animals a language that went beyond a few simple signals had clearly failed. Even chimpanzees, the cleverest of the higher primates, could not learn to speak, despite years of intensive efforts by devoted people. But it now appears that the chimpanzees' main problem was that they could not make the required sounds. Their vocal equipment is controlled by the emotional parts of their brains, so their screeches must remain involuntary. This does not mean, however, that they have no linguistic ability.

In 1966 the psychologists Allen and Beatrice Gardner of the University of Nevada began to train a one-year-old female chimpanzee, Washoe, in something that appeared more suitable – American Sign Language, the language of deaf-mutes. Chimpanzees obviously have plenty of manual dexterity. Within three years they had taught Washoe over eighty words; she began, as would any child, with 'come' and 'gimme'. Most surprising, the young chimpanzee spontaneously made hundreds of word-combinations of her own: 'hurry open', 'listen dog', 'you me go there' and others. By the time she was seven years old she could use nearly 200 signs. She had certainly reached the first stage of baby-talk. But it was not yet clear whether she had any concept of syntax – whether, for instance, she could make the distinction between 'listen dog', which she said when she heard a dog bark, and 'dog listen', should she ever want to express that thought.

Washoe's achievements soon became the subject of much argument. Throwing fuel into the fire, another experimenter began to communicate with a chimpanzee through plastic symbols. David Premack, of the University of California at Santa Barbara, originally wanted to find out how far a five-year-old chimpanzee named Sarah could go intellectually. He taught her about 130 words, each represented by a coloured plastic shape that clings to a magnetized board. To date, he has not been able to mark out the limits of her reasoning. Sarah uses her vocabulary to build original sentences and apparently can understand such concepts as 'colour of'. Having learned to associate the symbol for 'red' with an apple, and 'green' with grapes, she can apply these symbols to totally unfamiliar objects. On one occasion, she was asked to pick the proper symbols to describe a real apple (red, round) from several alternatives, did it correctly, and then was asked to describe the properties of the *symbol* for 'apple' (a blue triangle). Again she chose red and round – evidence, according to Premack, 'that the chimpanzee thinks of the word not as its literal form (blue plastic) but as the thing it represents (red apple)'. He further suspects that chimpanzees have an innate capacity for language, similar to man's. However, many linguists disagree vehemently. They point out that Sarah has never asked a question, and they refuse to call the chimpanzee's actions true language. In their opinion, her performance can be explained as a series of correct responses, learned much as B. F. Skinner's pigeons learn to play ping-pong through careful programming and reinforcement.

While these purely psychological arguments were going on, two scientists at Boston City Hospital discovered a sort of language lump in the human cortex – a slight but definite enlargement in part of the left temporal lobe, next to an area known to be involved in language. This was striking evidence of the asymmetry between the two hemispheres of man's brain. It had been known for more than a century that in most people only the left side of the brain controls speech. Damage in certain areas of the left hemisphere usually destroyed a person's ability to speak normally, though similar damage in the right hemisphere left speech unimpaired. But these differences in function were hardly reflected in any physical differences until Norman Geschwind and Walter Levitsky studied 100 normal brains and noticed a visible enlargement on the left side in sixty-five of them. More recently, other researchers have found a similar asymmetry even in the brains of infants who had died soon after birth. Though this evidence is still preliminary, it tends to reinforce the notion of man's unique and inborn competence for language.

Nevertheless, some scientists question the entire concept of the superiority of man's brain. John Lilly, a neurophysiologist and psychoanalyst who spent ten years studying the brains of dolphins, is convinced that their brains are superior to ours. Dolphins can communicate far more information through the right and left blowholes in their noses than we can communicate through our mouths, in the same period of time. They can even carry on two different conversations simultaneously – one in whistles and the other in clicks. They do this quite independently with the two halves of their brains. In addition, they produce ultrasounds through a separate echo-locating system. They are so far ahead of us in acoustic inputs and outputs that, Dr Lilly said, 'the problem is not for us to learn how they speak, but for them to learn how we speak. They can slow down their frequencies; we can't speed up and raise ours.'

In his well-equipped laboratory in the Virgin Islands Dr Lilly tried for years to teach some dolphins to speak English. He did get them to mimic a large number of sounds, despite the difference between their frequencies and ours. On several occasions he also saw them train one another. A week after he had taught a dolphin to produce the sounds for the numbers one to ten, for instance – a feat that required a good deal of effort and practice from the animal – he discovered that the dolphin in the adjacent tank could also count to ten. When he studied tapes of the conversations the two dolphins had been having at night, he heard instances of systematic coaching.

Language requires a critical brain-size, said Dr Lilly. There must be enough neurons to store, retrieve and compose words. The brains of humans reach the minimum necessary size (700 grams) at around six months of age. Among other mammals, only dolphins, whales and elephants have big enough brains; actually, their brains are often larger than ours. Lilly failed to find a really practical way to communicate with dolphins, however. He was working out a computerized method of transforming their acoustic world into three-dimensional pictures for men to see, when he closed down his lab. He had become aware of the ethical implications of his beliefs about dolphin intelligence, he explains. Once he realized how advanced the dolphins were, he could no longer 'run a concentration camp for advanced beings'.

Whether or not we are superior to all other living creatures, there are clear dangers in applying to men's brains techniques that have been developed through work with other species. In 1935 the Portuguese physician Egas Moniz heard a report about a female chimpanzee whose violent tantrums had been relieved by a brain operation. This gave him the idea of trying the same operation on human beings – and so frontal lobotomies were born. In the next two decades, until tranquillizers replaced them, these mutilating operations were performed on tens of thousands of mental patients to make them more manageable. The nerve fibres running from their frontal lobes to the deeper, more emotional parts of their brains were cut, blunting their minds. And although these patients did become less troublesome – they seemed to have stopped caring about anything – they also lost some of the very qualities that made them human: sensitivity, imagination, the ability to plan.

Current brain research can easily lend itself to equally hasty applications. Some scientists already advocate using brain surgery or 'peace pills' to deal with the problem of violence. Although most brain researchers are totally opposed to this suggestion, it is only one of many that can be expected as further knowledge about the brain pours out of the research labs.

The technology that will allow all kinds of brain manipulation is now within reach. What we still lack – desperately – is a fuller understanding of the effects of such intervention. Though sheltered by the skull and cushioned by fluids, like an egg yolk in its shell, the brain remains exceedingly vulnerable. Its delicacy and complexity inspire enormous respect. As I progressed with this book I began to tremble when my children fell and hit their heads. Watching the evening news, I shuddered at the sight of police cracking the heads of demonstrators. I realized that everything we do and think leaves a permanent imprint on our brains. And I worried about possible misuse of the current research.

Every advance in brain research leads to more questions about how, why, where and when the new techniques should be applied. Brain changes – and their regulation – will become

23

increasingly controversial, increasingly an issue for public debate.

Few people had heard of Einstein twenty years before the atomic bomb exploded over Hiroshima. The names of today's leading brain scientists are equally unknown, but by the end of this century, and perhaps sooner, their work will affect us as dramatically as Einstein's obscure equations.

2 Learning the language of the brain

In 1924 an Austrian psychiatrist, Hans Berger, discovered strange electrical signals coming from his son's brain. They were weak, but clearly detectable when Berger pasted two small pieces of silver foil on the fifteen-year-old's scalp, attached wires to them and connected them to a galvanometer. Furthermore, they followed a regular rhythm – he called it the 'alpha rhythm'. He could actually see this regularity when he recorded the galvanometer's oscillations on a roll of paper. Later on, working with other people, he noted that the rhythm broke whenever his subjects concentrated on arithmetic or other problems. Not only did people's brains emit signals, then, but these signals were directly related to their state of mind.

No one paid much attention to Berger's discovery at the time. A decade later, however, there was a flurry of excitement when the eminent physiologist Lord Adrian announced that he had confirmed Berger's findings. Suddenly brain waves became a sort of fad throughout Europe. Some people hoped these waves would enable them to read thoughts. Others expected to pick up distant brain waves on their own radio receivers – gadgets which themselves still seemed new and rather mysterious.

The fad soon ended, for neither the scientists' expectations nor the public's could be fulfilled. With the limited technology available to researchers in the 1930s the signals from the thousands of millions of cells in the brain proved almost impossible to unscramble. Their voltage was tiny – only a few hundred thousandths of a volt – and, even worse, the squiggles of the brain-wave records (called electroencephalograms, or E E Gs for short) all looked alike, at least in healthy people. They were 'disappointingly constant', Lord Adrian complained. E E Gs seemed to vary only with disease. Little by little, the E E G pioneers turned to medical applications. They used the waves to pinpoint brain tumours, injuries and other abnormalities, developing techniques that were of great value to surgeons, but learning little about the activity of normal brains. Those who persisted in trying to crack the language of the brain seemed to have reached a dead-end. Years of hard work produced few rewards, and several of these pioneers are now embittered men who wish they had been born decades later, in time to study the brain's chemistry rather than its electrical activity.

Yet they were right: the brain does speak a language of its own, and what it says reveals the inner state of man. Night and day the brain speaks, incessantly. When Descartes said, 'I think, therefore I am' he left out half of his self. Actually, his brain never slept, even when he did; it went on speaking even when he was unconscious. Since this chatter accompanied every breath he took, every eyeblink, every dream, every word, groan or response to heat or cold, *brain talk* was the ultimate proof of his existence.

The medical world has begun to recognize this fact. The need for organs to transplant is imperative in medicine today. To make sure that no one is robbed of his kidney or heart while he is still alive, doctors must fix the precise moment of death. Nowadays the E E G is the final arbiter in such matters. When its spikes or waves flatten out to a straight line – as in the unforgettable scene in the film *2001* – the brain has stopped talking, and this is the end.

Beyond these crude observations of noise versus silence, we remain much like illiterate primitives when faced with the complex language of the brain. But at least an alphabet exists, and scientists have begun to decipher some key words.

Their tools are high-speed digital computers, micro-miniaturized electronic equipment and new techniques made possible by a combination of the two. 'Looking at complicated waves with one's eyes, one can't see much,' explained Dr John Hanley, a British physiologist at the Space Biology Laboratory of UCLA's Brain Research Institute. 'It's like trying to study bacteria or viruses without a microscope. With computers, we can bring a physiological microscope to bear on the EEG signal.'

Recently scientists in this lab have shown that by running a chimpanzee's brain waves through a computer they can predict – within limited choices – what he will do next. They can determine whether a cat in a training programme is learning its lessons efficiently, or failing to learn at all. They can tell whether a person is calm or anxious, and whether certain questions shock him. They know whether a person is really sleeping or just pretending. They know when he is dreaming.

They can do all this by using their computers to analyse 'evoked responses' – the responses of the brain to specific signals such as light, sound or a problem to solve – rather than the meandering brain waves of people who are at rest. This allows them to tie certain kinds of responses to certain situations and then recognize them whenever they occur. In this way they are developing a whole vocabulary of brain states.

Mental telepathy, it was believed, would reveal a person's intimate thoughts or ideas. These researchers are producing a new form of telepathy that does not deal with the *content* of thoughts. Instead, it is attuned to emotions, to states such as sleep or semi-consciousness, and to subtle degrees of arousal and certain preparations for action of which the subject may not even be aware.

'Mental processes are rapid and changing,' said Dr W. Ross Adey, the Australian Director of the Space Biology Lab. 'We want to recognize states of consciousness that might last one second or less, as in rapid decision-making.' Other researchers had given up trying to pinpoint such states because of the large differences between subjects and because of technical difficulties. But Dr Adey's group attacked the problem in a big way. Working with 200 astronaut candidates, the scientists sat them down in a Houston laboratory for one hour and gave them tests of perception and learning interspersed with periods of quiet, while their brain waves were recorded from electrodes pasted at eighteen different places on their heads. A high-speed computer then averaged the output from each of these eighteen locations, for each of fifty men, during more than twelve specific situations. The result was a series of clearly discernible patterns. For example, when the men were tested for 'auditory vigilance' and were told to listen for three tones that would ring in a row, their brain-wave patterns were quite different from those seen during visual tasks. 'There is an E E G signature for each state,' Dr Adey said. 'Our study established for the first time that common factors clearly categorize E E G records in such a population for a series of specified behavioural states.'

Dr Adey is probably the most adventurous E E G researcher active today. He tackles problems of moon travel, brain physiology and undersea exploration with equal energy. At times he sounds like an engineer, but actually he is both a surgeon and a professor of physiology.

His work has its detractors, however; at a meeting in Washington, D.C., of the American E E G Society, some of the more conservative members challenged Dr Adey's work. 'These are very beautiful instrumental techniques,' declared the eminent Dr Reginald Bickford, a professor of neurosciences at the University of California at San Diego. 'I am impressed with the electronic data. There is a problem, however: the incredible ability of muscles around the head to pull your leg. It's hard enough to get a record that isn't full of artifacts, even in a laboratory. But when people are activated, there are many changes of nuance in their muscles. You can produce nice rhythmic waves with eye movements. Chewing produces spike waves. And movements of the tongue – you don't really know when people are moving their tongues! I feel the computers have got ahead of our knowledge of the E E G. Short of cutting off people's tongues and ripping out their eyeballs . . .'

He was interrupted by Dr Adey, who marched up to the microphone. 'This isn't even old wine in *new* bottles!' he told Dr Bickford heatedly. 'You present such remarks every year. Any scientific explanation to be valid must be both necessary and sufficient. Are artifacts *so* distorting that we cannot use the data? Every piece of data that goes into the computer has been carefully checked so artifacts are not significant.'

Since no one is about to insert electrodes into the brains of human beings just to settle this point, it remains in doubt. EEG signals from the surface of the scalp do include many confusing elements. With animals, however, Dr Adey's group has achieved far more clear-cut results. It has implanted electrodes well under the cortex of cats and chimpanzees, placing them in several deep structures, including the hippocampus, a small sea-horse-shaped structure, about three centimetres long, which is involved in memory and learning. Then it has analysed the resulting EEGs on a computer and developed ways of foretelling whether an animal that has learned a certain skill will make a mistake within the next few seconds.

This is the beginning of scientific mind-reading – or perhaps a step beyond telepathy and into prophecy.

To understand the way it works one can follow the Space Biology Lab's experiments with Jerry, a chimpanzee who learned to play noughts-and-crosses. Noughts-and-crosses is a fairly complex game – children seldom learn to play it before the age of five, and among animals only chimpanzees are considered clever enough to do so. Jerry learned it slowly but well, receiving banana pellets as rewards for correct moves. Electrodes had been implanted in several parts of his brain, but the team did not begin to study his EEGs until after he had mastered the game. Then, as a sort of warm-up exercise, it tried to tell from Jerry's brain waves whether he was merely watching the board to see what his opponent would do, or whether he was preparing to make a move of his own. These two states were quite different, it turned out, and the team soon learned to recognize their characteristics. 'This way we knew that we weren't just studying attention,' explained Dr Hanley. Next the scientists attempted to distinguish between two forms of preparation for action: the kind leading to a correct move, and the kind leading to error. That is, they tried to tell whether the chimp was making the right or wrong decision. To avoid ambiguity, they ignored all the preliminary moves that came before he had a chance to complete a row, and all the times when Jerry did not respond at all. The chimp's moves were rated 'correct' only when he had an opportunity to complete a row and actually did so. 'Incorrect' meant that he had missed this opportunity by selecting the wrong panel. Again these distinctions became clear from Jerry's brain-wave records alone. When he made a mistake, Dr Hanley pointed out, 'it wasn't inattention, since he did respond. Maybe it was a very special kind of inattention – we really don't know. All we know is that his brain had to be in a certain condition for him to get it right.'

Suppose a man were given several tasks to do, all of them quite simple, and for some reason made an error on one of them – the situation would be the same. In all likelihood, his mind would simply have strayed for a moment. Since the game was easy for Jerry, the chimpanzee rarely made a mistake. When he did, however, the researchers were surprised to find that all the parameters of his EEG showed *more* activity than before a correct move. This was especially true of activity in the theta frequency (3 to 7 cycles per second, as compared with the faster alpha rhythm, which is between 8 and 12 cycles per second) from the thalamus, a central processing area at the top of the brain stem. 'Perhaps,' thought Dr Hanley, 'it is easier to do it right.' No one is quite sure yet how to interpret these findings.

The predictions were extremely reliable. After Jerry's individual EEG pattern for correct or incorrect moves had been established, his moves could be forecast accurately 99 per cent of the time. His brain waves told the tale well before he acted: usually the pattern was clear as much as seventeen or eighteen seconds in advance.

A margin of this kind confers enormous powers of control. This will become particularly obvious when scientists learn to make accurate predictions without opening up their subjects' skulls – when they can get all the information they need from electrodes on the surface of the head. (With present technology, EEGs from Jerry's scalp allowed accurate predictions of his moves only 70 per cent of the time.) Then, armed with fore-knowledge of a person's mental state, teachers and controllers of all kinds will be able to judge intentions as well as deeds.

By monitoring a pilot's brain waves at critical times, for in-stance, one could vastly improve his performance. He would be warned not to start some dangerous manoeuvre until his mental condition was just right. This would prevent the sort of 'human error' that is responsible for so many accidents. In education, the precious seventeen or eighteen seconds' leeway could help teachers to present their material more efficiently, particularly in computerized instruction. It could give students a euphoric sense of brilliance as they pass all tests with glowing colours, thanks to a new form of 'errorless learning'. Suppose that a child were given a problem to do, and that his brain waves showed he was about to make a mistake. A signal would then alert the teacher or the computer. During the next eighteen seconds, the computer would have plenty of time to re-phrase the question, switch to an easier problem, or stop altogether. Errorless learning of this kind would certainly reduce a student's frustration and might be especially useful for children with learning difficulties.

'Are there optimal brain states for learning?' asked Dr Hanley. 'Certainly there are sub-optimal states – after a heavy lunch, for instance. As an extreme case, learning is difficult dur-ing an epileptic seizure! Therefore, there may be optimal states, too – but when? Though they may be very fleeting, they may occur more often during certain times of day. Perhaps there are periodicities in our ability to learn, just as there are periodic-ities in many body functions, circadian rhythms. When we dis-cover what they are, we can capitalize on them.'

31

The scientists at the Space Biology Lab seem most comfortable with this idea of capitalizing on certain brain waves that people naturally produce. They want to turn serendipity into a science. Only a few of them wish to *increase* the brain's production of 'good' states, rather than catch them on the fly.

Thus Dr Rochelle Gavalas, a young psychologist, stands out for her startling plan to make animals produce different brainwave patterns simply by changing the electric fields around their heads. 'I know this sounds like science fiction,' she says apologetically, 'but it may not be so far off.'

As she points out, we are all surrounded by very weak electric currents that flow out of wires in the walls, telephone lines, radios, tvs, fluorescent lights and other appliances – currents so weak that we cannot feel them, but which exist nevertheless. Conceivably, they could match, interfere with, or enhance the weak electric activity in our brains. Little is known about the effects of ordinary household current, which is generated at approximately 50 cycles per second. But research on lower frequencies is progressing rapidly. Dr Gavalas and her associates have been studying the effects of very low frequency fields: 7 cycles per second. 'We picked this frequency because it corresponds to the upper range of the brain's theta waves,' she explained. Theta waves, perhaps the most interesting and mysterious rhythms in the brain, have been associated with memory and deep reverie as well as, paradoxically, anxiety. Dr Gavalas wanted to find out whether macaque monkeys would produce more or fewer theta waves of their own when their heads were placed in an electric field of theta frequency, and whether their behaviour would also change.

First she implanted electrodes into the cortex and deeper brain structures of three pigtailed macaque monkeys. Next she taught the monkeys to push a panel at five-second intervals – a period of time which they had to determine for themselves. (For each correct response, they earned a squirt of apple juice.) When the monkeys were trained to perform regularly, she placed large metal plates on both sides of their heads, fifteen inches apart, and sent a weak electric current between the plates. After a while, the monkeys began to respond more rapidly. They pushed the panel half a second sooner than before, as if their reactions had accelerated or their sense of time had changed. When experimenters in other labs exposed human beings to currents of equally low frequencies, they observed a similar speeding up. Why this should happen is not yet clear. Because the monkeys had implanted electrodes, however, Dr Gavalas was able to see that there was a distinct increase in the theta waves coming from their hippocampus. This seemed to mirror the electric current outside their heads. She finds this increased production of theta waves encouraging enough to ask, 'Can one expedite learning by superimposing external electric fields?' The answer will be yes, she believes. Someday, students may 'turn on' with weak electric currents to improve their powers of learning. They may use specific frequencies for different goals – one frequency for committing things to memory, perhaps, and others to achieve peak performance in music, art or mathematics, which presumably involve different brain structures and different kinds of electric activity.

It has always been difficult to judge the efficiency of anyone's brain. Too many factors can cloud the picture – the subject's anxiety, for instance, or his unfamiliarity with the middle-class culture on which most intelligence tests are based. Any test that uses language must have a built-in bias, since language styles differ according to social class.

Working on the theory that all people with normal vision are exposed to light in approximately the same way, regardless of their education or social class, a Canadian psychologist, Dr John Ertl, recently devised a culture-free test of what he calls 'neural efficiency'. This simply shows, on an EEG, how rapidly a person's brain responds to a flash of light. As Dr Ertl emphasizes, it does not measure intelligent behaviour but the underlying speed of mental reactions on which all intelligence depends. Conversation, reading, writing and rapport with the

B

examiner are all unnecessary – the subject just sits there, with electrodes pasted on his head, while a light flashes 100 times at random and a computer averages out his brain's reactions to it. When Dr Ertl tested 573 Ottawa schoolchildren of different ages and social class, he found large variations in the speed of their responses. The ten slowest children required more than twice as much time to react to the light as the ten fastest ones, who also scored higher on standard I Q tests. However, those children who suffered from language difficulties or other handicaps, such as nervousness, scored much lower on the I Q tests than they did on Ertl's test of neural efficiency.

It seems typical of the current research on brain waves that this test bypasses a person's actual behaviour and concentrates on how information is processed in his brain. Such research offers a rare glimpse into what happens *before* a person makes a move, speaks or even thinks, in the accepted meaning of the word. Even subliminal impressions, so fleeting that one is not consciously aware of them, may be reflected in an E E G.

This is a frightening breach of privacy. As we learn more about the language of the brain, the applications of this research will multiply. Already, some scientists are speculating about the possibility of using E E Gs, combined with computers, as a new, ominously prescient lie-detection device.

At the California Institute of Technology, for instance, Dr Derek Fender, an English physicist-turned-biologist, has developed a method with which he hopes to trace various mental operations as they progress from one area of the brain to the next. The air-conditioned helmet that he designed for this purpose has forty-nine electrodes – about four times the number normally used for E E Gs. He needs so many because it takes at least nine electrodes to zero in on the source of a single brain wave, he says. To locate two source-points accurately requires at least thirty electrodes at strategic spots on the scalp, since the waves from the two sources may be intermingled by the time they reach the surface of the head. With the full forty-nine electrodes, and extensive work from a large computer, he can follow some of the lightning-swift operations in the brain as a person responds to light or noise.

Looking straight at me, Dr Fender said, 'You are watching my face as I speak, and your ears are hearing a train of sound waves.' At that point, a bell happened to ring in the university hall. 'Your brain identifies these sounds quite clearly,' Dr Fender continued. 'One set is from my mouth, the other comes from the bell. You correlate them in time and space. Well,' he said significantly, 'we can now pick out the part of the brain that does such correlations.'

In his experiments, Dr Fender studied the brain waves of twenty-seven volunteers as they were exposed to light flashes and, sometimes, simultaneous clicking sounds. If the clicks came from the same point in space as the flash, three areas in the brain would generate waves. One would be the area that analyses visual images; the second, the area that analyses sound signals. 'And then I would see further activity up here, in the parietal area [Dr Fender pointed to the back of his head] as the brain worked out that the click and the flash had come from the same source.'

If noise and light clearly came from different sources, there would be no integrative activity. But if a person's brain did begin to integrate the two signals in the parietal area, the next step – still followed by a fascinated Dr Fender – would be some activity in the frontal motor area as it prepared to send neural messages to the eye muscles to get them focused on the right spot. The scientist was thus in the privileged position of being able to predict that a few milliseconds later the volunteer would turn his eyes towards the source of light and sound.

'You could probably work out a lie-detector based on similar principles,' Dr Fender said. 'Now, this is not part of my research, you understand – I've only tried it out on three people, and it's more like a form of play for me. But near the speech centre in the brain there is an area that prepares the neural messages that drive the muscles associated with speech. I can identify the activity in that area that is associated with the word "yes" and with the word "no", *whether you say it out loud or not.*' This statement nearly left me speechless, but Dr Fender continued confidently. 'You see, the actions of the tongue, teeth, etcetera, are quite different for these two words. Naturally, the patterns of the nerve signals that go out to make these two words will be different as well. These patterns are formed long before the word ever reaches the vocalizing level. So if it's just a question of "yes" or "no", I can tell from your brain what the answer will be – even if you're a completely unco-operative subject.'

Of course, each person's brain, being unique, will prepare to utter the word 'yes' in a slightly different way, though some features would probably be common to all people. An interrogator would need some experience with a subject's individual wave patterns before he could read these thoughts accurately. 'But possibly in casual conversation one could get the characteristic pattern of "yes" and "no" for an individual,' suggested Dr Fender. 'This pattern *cannot* change.' The only salvation for an 'unco-operative subject', then, would be to avoid even *thinking* of any words he had spoken before.

Is it right for anyone to gain such intimate knowledge of another person's mind? This kind of snooping seems a dangerous pastime, even if it is still impractical. (It took Dr Fender's powerful computer as long as forty-four minutes to figure out what had happened during a quarter of a second of activity in one man's brain.) Primitive as they are, the various attempts at scientific mind reading do offer potential tools for prediction, as well as revelation. And when one can predict something, one can often control it – intercept it, change it or turn it off entirely.

Some scientists yearn for such control; the majority do not. Ross Adey's group, for the most part, is simply trying to learn the language of the brain. But the possibility of exerting power over the brain is a great temptation for many people.

Among the activists, there are two main streams: one group of researchers has been changing the brain's activity by force, opening up the skulls of animals and sometimes humans, to implant electrodes or chemicals. A totally different group of scientists, more interested in individual freedom, has started teaching people to produce certain mental states at will, using nothing more formidable than scalp E E Gs and computers that provide instant information, a technique called 'bio-feedback'.

3 Remote control of the brain: through pain and pleasure

The most frightening visions of brain control involve people walking about with little black boxes inside their skulls, slaves to electronic orders from a dictator far away. 'Push-button people' they have been called – just the thing to turn a whole generation of students off science.

Such visions are rather naïve, since they assume that one could actually send complex messages to a person's brain cells ('Now go and murder so-and-so') or that dictators don't have far more practical means of controlling human behaviour. The most sophisticated electronic equipment in the world could not transmit thoughts directly to the brain. Besides, brain surgery is intricate and time-consuming. Finding the specific brain cells that control even the simplest motor act is exceedingly difficult. A dictator intent on making people obey him would do much better with mind-altering drugs, threats or brute force.

Nevertheless, it's true that little black boxes can be implanted into human brains – scores of people have had them, supposedly for therapeutic reasons. Limited kinds of orders can be transmitted to the brain from a distance; these are orders to electrodes in a man's brain, telling them to stimulate certain cells with a weak electric current. And, most significant, there is now a growing possibility that brain implants may some day be used for various kinds of training or restraint.

At present, brain stimulation is used mostly for diagnosis. In some neurological centres fine-needle electrodes are inserted into the brains of hundreds of patients as a prelude to further surgery, either to record the activity of certain areas or to stimulate them – for example, to help doctors locate cells that set off severe epileptic attacks. Brain-stimulation experiments are never performed on normal people. At times, though, surgeons have explored the brains of patients whose skulls they had opened for other reasons. Thus Canada's great neurosurgeon Dr Wilder Penfield made use of every opportunity that presented itself in his practice. With his patients' consent, he would stimulate selected spots in their brains during operations and record everything the patient did or said. He considered it his duty to science. In this way, he mapped out areas of the brain involved in speech, memory and language, as well as in specific sensations or movements.

This was possible because the brain, unlike any other part of the body, cannot feel what is being done to it. There are no touch or pain receptors in the brain. The organ that registers all the pleasures and pains of existence does not even know when its own tissue is being penetrated or cut. Once a surgeon has removed a piece of skull and some of the brain's outer covering under anaesthesia, he is free to explore the pink-grey jelly as he pleases: wide-awake and conscious, the patient won't feel it. Nor can he feel a foreign object placed amidst his brain cells. As a result, many researchers have taken to leaving instruments inside the brain to carry on their work over a long period of time, much as explorers have left instruments on the moon.

Such objects can stay in the brain for months or even years. Generally they are left in experimental animals, but occasionally an adventurous surgeon will cement electrodes into the brain of a patient as well, though there are serious questions about the safety of leaving them there until better and lighter electrodes are developed.

Today we are on the verge of entirely new uses for brain implants because of two discoveries made in the 1950s and a new link with computers. Together, these may make the little black boxes much too valuable to ignore, despite their difficulties and the natural horror they inspire.

The discoveries involve what really happens when we feel pleasure or pain from any source. Though we may think our happiness is caused by love, sex, food, music or good news, it is actually produced by a thin stream of cells in the centre of our brain. In these cells lies the ultimate reward for our activities. Adjacent cells hold the ultimate punishment. And both sets can be stimulated with electrodes.

For psychologists, this means a chance to develop a powerful teaching device. Tie electrodes in the brain's own reward or punishment centres to a computer that has been programmed to keep track of some specific behaviour, and you have immediacy, repetition, speed – all the elements of a fiendishly efficient system, the most effective form of conditioning known to date.

Such computer-linked implants might become an integral part of the brain's functioning. They could be used for training or re-training. They would alter personalities, produce certain kinds of behaviour, make permanent changes that go far beyond the control of a single physical movement. What their ultimate consequences would be we cannot yet forsee.

Paddy is a chimpanzee who lives in a laboratory at Yale University. He has had 100 electrodes implanted in his brain for years. A small box of electronic equipment protrudes from the top of his head, where it has been permanently attached with dental cement. The box is called a 'stimoceiver', because it can both stimulate various parts of Paddy's brain, according to radioed instructions, and receive his E E Gs, which it then transmits some distance by radio. Wherever Paddy goes and whatever he does, the stimoceiver is always on the alert.

In a room nearby, a computer stands watch. Its job is to pick out some strange spikes, or spindles, in the brain waves produced by the amygdalas – small bundles of nerve cells in the limbic system – on both sides of Paddy's brain. These spindles come every few seconds, especially when Paddy is aroused by meeting friends, smelling new odours or being groomed by another chimpanzee.

And now the experiment begins.

As Paddy approaches a friendly chimpanzee, the stimoceiver on his skull radios his E E G to the computer, which recognizes a burst of spindles from his right amygdala. Immediately the computer radios back instructions to stimulate another area in Paddy's brain, in the right reticular formation, which causes Paddy to wince. It is like a sudden spanking, but all in the chimpanzee's brain, and it happens in a flash.

More than a thousand times, in the next two hours, the computer lightly punishes Paddy for every burst of spindles from his right amygdala. It pays no attention to the left side of Paddy's brain. At the end of the session, the spindles from his right amygdala are reduced to half their usual rate.

The following day, Paddy's amygdala remembers its lessons and still spindles at the reduced rate. This does not prevent the computer from going back to work and dishing out its punishment for every single spindle. Within six days, the spindles on the right side of Paddy's brain are almost completely wiped out. Meanwhile, his left amygdala goes on spindling as before, some 1,000 times an hour – a beautiful demonstration of specific control.

It takes Paddy two full weeks to return to normal. At that point, the experimenters decide to block the spindles on both sides of the brain. The computer begins to punish right and left, wherever there is an offending spindle. And again the spindles are practically eliminated within six days. (Actually his right amygdala is tamed much more rapidly, since it remembers what it learned before.) But as the spindles disappear, Paddy becomes strangely quiet. Though he was a lively chimp before the experiment, now he just sits in his chair, performing whatever tasks are required of him, and barely moving. He doesn't look at the food pellets that are given him as rewards; nor, in most cases, does he eat them. He doesn't dare be aroused by anything. For weeks after the end of this experiment, Paddy remains as humble as a whipped dog.

It's now almost a hundred years since two German scientists, Gustav Fritsch and Eduard Hitzig, gave the first demonstrations of how electrical stimulation of the brain could control behaviour. Very systematically, they applied a weak electric current to various areas of the cerebral cortex – the brain's outermost layer – and recorded what happened to their subjects, dogs. In most cases, since the dogs were anaesthetized, nothing happened. But all across one area of the cortex, a wide band extending from one side of the head to the other, the application of the current provoked physical movement. When they ran current to one point on this band, the dog would lift a leg; another point, and his mouth would twitch. Soon it was found that other animals – cats, monkeys, chimpanzees – also had what came to be called a motor area in their cortex. Later work revealed a sensory area, which received sensations of touch, temperature and position from all over the body; a visual area, which processed information from the eyes; an auditory area; and so on. Much has been learnt about the cortex, though vast areas of it remain as mysterious as those stretches of unexplored territory on ancient maps.

No one ventured deeper into the brain until 1924, when a Swiss physiologist, Walter Hess, discovered the tremendous importance of the hypothalamus. Hess, who later won the Nobel Prize, began by inserting thin tubes into the brain stems of cats and injecting small amounts of chemicals through them. This produced extraordinary changes in the animals' behaviour, as if he had hit the centre of their emotions. Startled, Hess decided to stimulate the same area electrically. Using thin but rigid electric wires that were completely insulated except at their tips, he ran a weak electric current to the cats' hypothalami. This, too, produced dramatic changes of even greater variety. By stimulating one spot, he could make a cat behave 'as if threatened by a dog', he reported. 'It spits, snorts or growls . . . its pupils widen . . . its ears lie back, or move back and forth to frighten the non-existent enemy.' One cat was so enraged that it attacked Hess. Stimulation at other spots, only millimetres away, changed the cats' rate of breathing and blood pressure, made them eat, drink or vomit, aroused them sexually, or made them sleep.

If Hess had done nothing more than sketch the functions of the hypothalamus in this way, he would have earned his reputation as one of the giants of brain research. The hypothalamus is now recognized as so powerful and complex that it has been called 'a brain within a brain'. It regulates the entire autonomic nervous system, and thus the body's internal environment, including its temperature, chemical balance and appetites, as well as the emotions.

But Hess is also the father of brain implants. He mistrusted the existing techniques of brain exploration, in which researchers held their electrodes in their own hands. If moving an electrode one millimetre could produce such extreme differences in behaviour, the hand-held style was much too inaccurate. It also required that the subjects be physically restrained or anaesthetized throughout the entire experiment so that they would lie absolutely still, making any normal reaction impossible. Instead, Hess positioned his electrodes inside the cats' brains and left them there, attached to a fixed terminal on the scalp. He showed that after recovering from this operation, the cats behaved normally. Then he attached flexible wires to the terminals on their heads and connected these to instruments suspended from the ceiling, allowing the cats to move about on a leash. He could now stimulate their brains as often as he wished, always at exactly the same spot, while the cats were active and conscious. Furthermore, after he had finished his tests, he could study the brains under a microscope to determine precisely where the electrodes had been.

Nobody could doubt Hess' evidence: when he stimulated certain parts of the cats' hypothalami, the cats reacted angrily. But did this mean that the cats actually *felt* angry? Most scientists claimed it did not. Although they knew that electrical

43

stimulation of the cortex could produce physical movements, these were considered purely mechanical responses. Emotions were something else again – far more private, closer to the soul. When one is angry, the whole person is angry. Surely the emotions could not be localized or triggered in the brain as simply as the movement of a toe. Therefore, his colleagues said, what Hess produced with his brain stimulation was only 'sham' rage or fear – only the physical manifestations of emotion, not the emotion itself.

In the early 1950s, however. Hess appeared to be vindicated. By then thinner electrodes, many of which could be implanted simultaneously in a single brain, and better techniques to implant them had led to a new burst of experiments with brain stimulation. Suddenly one group of researchers at Yale University reported finding some brain areas where stimulation produced either fear or pain, while a young American working at McGill University in Montreal discovered that he could produce artificial pleasure.

The Yale experiment involved some very hungry cats with electrodes in their brains. Offered food, they ran towards it, but as soon as they began to eat, a current stimulated certain points in their thalamus, which is just above the hypothalamus, and other deep structures. The cats dropped the food immediately, as if stung by it, and retreated. After a few attempts, they avoided the food altogether, despite their hunger. Equally hungry cats that were stimulated in different parts of the brain seemed momentarily distracted from the food, but went right back to it a second later.

If starved animals learn to shun food because it is coupled with a certain kind of brain stimulation, that stimulation must be powerfully unpleasant. There can be nothing 'sham' about it! Thus Dr José Delgado, the physiologist, working with the psychologists Warren Roberts and Neal Miller, demonstrated in 1954 that real pain can be produced by electrical stimulation of the brain.

They also showed that brain pain is a most efficient spur to learning. This led to a long line of experiments, including Dr Delgado's successful attempt to make Paddy turn off certain brain waves from his amygdala. Paddy's pain was not 'sham', either, but Dr Delgado insists that at the low intensity of current he used (.5 milliamps) the stimulation was not really disturbing.

Dr Delgado is a controversial Spanish-born professor of physiology who seems to enjoy giving dramatic demonstrations of his latest gadgets. He once made the front page of the *New York Times* by stopping a bull in mid-charge in a Cordova bullring. As photographers watched, he faced an enormous bull. He waved a red cape, just like a matador. But when the beast charged, he did not lure it to his side. Instead, he pressed a button on a small radio transmitter that he carried in his left hand, and suddenly the bull ground to a halt, raising a cloud of dust. Actually Dr Delgado had run no risk: he had implanted electrodes into the bull's caudate nucleus, a subcortical area that inhibits all motor activity, and he knew that whenever he pressed the button the bull would be forced to stop. This exploit did not please his colleagues, many of whom considered it too sensational and unscholarly. But the impressive display of power over a wild beast fascinated the public.

Dr Delgado has also developed techniques for absolute control over monkeys. By stimulating different spots in their brains, he can make them perform like puppets; eat a thousand times more than they normally would, yawn, wake up or go through elaborate routines, surprising sequences that apparently result from the individual monkey's previous experience and the fact that the cerebral organization of monkeys is more stereotyped than man's. Dr Delgado tells how he made one female monkey carry out the following sequence 20,000 times in a row: she would stop whatever she was doing, change her facial expression, turn her head to the right, stand upright, circle to the right, walk on two feet with perfect balance, climb a pole, come down, growl, threaten and attack any subordinate monkey, suddenly become peaceful again, and approach the rest of the group in a friendly manner. The whole sequence took ten to fourteen seconds. It was always performed in the same order, but with some changes in detail according to circumstances.

Dr Delgado can also topple monkey dictators, or increase their power. Monkey societies are normally autocratic, he explains. One animal takes over as boss of the group. In one experiment, Dr Delgado stimulated the boss monkey's brain to make him more aggressive. The boss then chased and bit his subordinates, especially his nearest rival, the second-ranking male, but always spared 'the little female who was his favourite partner'. This aggression merely strengthened his position as boss.

A sadder fate was in store for Ali, the bad-tempered chief of another monkey colony. Ali was universally feared by his subordinates, who huddled in a corner while he lorded over two thirds of the cage. He occasionally glared at them, but they hardly dared steal a glance at him. When Dr Delgado stimulated his caudate nucleus, however, Ali lost the power to be aggressive. His expression changed, and the other monkeys in the cage began to move about freely, edging closer to him. After a while, they actually crowded around him without fear whenever the current was on. Then Dr Delgado installed a new lever on the cage wall – a lever that triggered the stimulation of Ali's brain by radio. Soon a female monkey named Elsa discovered that when she pressed this lever, Ali became quite harmless. Every time Ali threatened her, she ran to the lever and pressed it. She did the same whenever he threatened any other monkey. Elsa thus became the Joan of Arc of her colony, the defender of the oppressed, cutting off Ali's strength whenever he tried to assert himself as boss again.

In his book *Physical Control of the Mind: Toward a Phycho-civilized Society* Dr Delgado describes how a patient with electrodes in his brain was forced to close his hand into a fist every time the current passed through a certain spot. The patient did not seem to mind having to make a fist, which he knew was involuntary. But when Dr Delgado asked him to try to keep his fingers extended during the next stimulation, he couldn't do it. As Dr Delgado reports, the patient then said, 'I guess, doctor, that your electricity is stronger than my will.'

Though his electricity was indeed strong, Dr Delgado remained limited by the primitive state of knowledge about how the brain functions. When he placed his electrodes in the man's brain, he could not have predicted what the stimulation would do. From the electrodes' placement he knew only that he would produce some motor activity, probably involving the man's hand. He could not have *planned* to make the man close his hand. Nor did he know ahead of time that he would force another patient to turn his head to the side, as if looking for something, every time the current was turned on. Once he produced these reactions, however, he could make the patients do them over and over again.

'The interesting fact was that the patient considered the evoked activity spontaneous, and always offered a reasonable explanation for it,' Dr Delgado wrote. When the patient turned his head, Dr Delgado asked him what he was doing. 'I am looking for my slippers,' the man said one time. On other occasions he replied, 'I heard a noise,' 'I am restless,' or 'I was looking under the bed.' This implies not only control over the man's behaviour, but the power to make him think that he willed what, in fact, was electrically forced on him.

Dr Delgado also describes how an otherwise reserved thirty-year-old woman reacted to stimulation in one part of her brain: when he pressed the button, she 'openly expressed her fondness for the therapist (who was new to her), kissed his hands, and talked about her immense gratitude for what was being done for her'.

Such power is frightening enough. Yet what really worries liberals – and some of Dr Delgado's fellow scientists – is not so much what he does as what he says about it. In his book Dr Delago urges the government to make 'conquering of the human mind' a national goal. He foresees a new age in which the brains of human beings can be regulated from a distance, as easily as one can now open or close the doors of a garage by pushing a button in one's car. Natural evolution is too slow, he says. We will have to intervene directly in the fate of man by implanting 'cerebral pacemakers', similar to cardiac pacemakers, which would maintain people's mental stability at all times and thus preserve peace.

An epileptic equipped with such a pacemaker might go about his business without fear of having a seizure. Whenever his brain waves showed signs of an impending attack, his pacemaker would alert a computer, which would trigger stimulation in an inhibitory area of his brain and prevent the attack. The patient might never know it happened, as the stimulation might be below the level of conscious perception.

Brain implants might well prove acceptable in clear-cut medical cases like this one, especially if the epilepsy could not be controlled by any other means, and if safer electrodes were developed. Some doctors might also go along with Dr Delgado's prescription of cerebral pacemakers to prevent violent behaviour, at least in certain extreme cases (see Chapter 9). But when he speaks of using implants to treat such widespread ills as anxiety, fear and obsessive behaviour he makes all of us possible candidates for brain stimulation.

Dr Delgado's real significance lies outside philosophy, however, in the realm of technological advances. Nobody has used the spin-offs from the space race more fruitfully. When micro-miniaturized radio receivers became available he attached them to the kind of brain implants invented by Walter Hess and gave his subjects total freedom of movement, making it possible to stimulate their brains by remote control. Later on, he replaced the radio receivers with tiny two-way radios, creating the stimoceiver. Now he is deeply involved in three projects: embedding the stimoceiver inside his subject's body, to hide it under the skin; linking the stimoceiver to a computer, as he did with Paddy; and developing a whole new line of chemical implants.

The stimoceivers he has used so far have been external, he

explains. 'This is always a possible source of infection, and a hindrance to grooming. But now we will fit the instrument inside the body. I will use a new, transdermal stimulator,' he told me. He opened a small box he had taken out of his pocket. It contained a round, flat piece of metal, rather like an outsized coin, with some designs on it. He handed me the box and a jeweller's magnifying-glass. 'Look at it,' he said. 'This is a next-generation transdermal.' I peered through the glass, and the designs on the coin turned into intricate printed circuits. 'We've started using it with gibbons,' he said. 'There are no wires, nothing piercing the skin, nothing visible. Then we can telemeter instructions transdermally.'

Some time ago, Dr Delgado exhibited his inventions during a meeting of the American Psychiatric Association. The passing psychiatrists seemed highly interested in his exhibit of stimoceivers and his film of a monkey being tamed by a chemical injected deep in its brain through another gadget, a 'dialytrode'. Some of them did a double take and asked if Dr Delgado wasn't the man who stopped the bull. 'Where are the bulls?' inquired one psychiatrist. Dr Delgado's assistant shook his head mournfully. 'Everybody is asking for the bulls today,' he muttered. 'I think the experiment was very unfortunate.' Undaunted, Dr Delgado went on explaining the virtues of the dialytrode.

This, he said, is 'perhaps the most important thing for the future. We are establishing a two-way chemical communication with specific areas of the brain.' Up to now, to investigate brain chemistry, 'it was necessary to kill your experimental subject'. But a few years ago, his lab began to develop a system of dialytrodes – two thin tubes ending in a dialysis bag, implanted permanently anywhere in the brain, through which an experimenter can inject chemicals and collect chemical information from the brain. As the name implies, dialytrodes can also stimulate the brain electrically and record electrical activity, thus doubling as electrodes, though they are somewhat thicker. 'Now we have a method to investigate brain chemistry in live animals,' he said, 'to study the side actions of some drugs, or the release of neurohumours at certain times.'

As Dr Delgado sees it, the main barrier to using brain implants in human beings is the 'cosmetic' aspect. 'For humans, you can't have these plugs in the head,' he said. 'Everything must be under the skin.' Fortunately, a new transdermal dialytrode is nearly ready. This will include two small terminal bags, one for each tube, to be placed under the scalp at the outlet of the implanted tubes. It will then be a simple matter for a doctor to inject fluid into one bag, or withdraw it from the other, by means of a hypodermic needle.

'Then we can inject drugs locally into any area of the brain,' Dr Delgado said with satisfaction. 'We can block certain areas functionally – that's far more conservative than surgery, as we don't need to destroy anything. We can also use synthetic spinal fluid, circulate it through the dialysis bag, and collect chemical information on what happens inside the brain.'

Dr Delgado hopes to use both of his transdermal gadgets – the stimoceiver and the dialytrode – in human beings soon, to block the perception of pain in otherwise hopeless cases. He remains very interested in pain and its prevention.

The Yale group's original work on pain centres was soon overshadowed by the far more exciting discovery that there were areas in the brain where electric stimulation produced pleasure. This came to light accidentally, in 1953, when Dr James Olds noticed the odd behaviour of a white rat.

Dr Olds, a young American psychologist, had come to Canada to work under Donald Hebb, a pioneer in the study of how the brain processes information. He was just beginning an experiment on the effects of brain stimulation on animals when his very first rat surprised him. The rat had a pair of wires deep in its brain, through which Dr Olds stimulated it every time it entered a specific corner of a large maze. Naturally Dr Olds expected that this would teach the rat to stay away from that particular spot. But the rat – perversely, it seemed – appeared to like that corner, and after a few minutes it came back for more. In fact, Dr Olds found that he could make the rat move in any direction he liked merely by turning the current on whenever the animal took a step in the right direction. However, he could not repeat this trick with the next few rats that he and Dr Peter Milner, another student of Dr Hebb, tried to stimulate in the same way.

When this strange rat was killed, Dr Olds saw at once that there had been a mistake: although the electrode was supposed to end in the rat's midbrain, it had landed a trifle too high, next to the hypothalamus – close to the areas investigated by Dr Hess. He guessed that he had discovered a brain centre of 'reward' – this was as close as he got to calling it 'pleasure'. He never learned precisely where the electrode had landed, however, because the brain was badly damaged, having been prepared for examination by an amateur. To hit the right place again and see how far it extended, he and Dr Milner would have to make a highly detailed map.

It is of course impossible to know how animals feel, but the psychologist B. F. Skinner had devised a technique to measure – if not explain – some kinds of motivation: the famous Skinner box, in which experimental animals can be given food pellets or other rewards every time they perform a particular action, like pushing a lever. As long as rewards are unavailable, the animals push the lever only occasionally, perhaps five to ten times an hour; but when they discover that they can earn something they like, their activity rate shoots up in a measurable way. This was the system Dr Olds and Dr Milner decided to use in mapping out different areas of the rats' brains. They inserted electrodes in various places and then, ingeniously, allowed the rats to stimulate their own brains by means of a foot pedal connected to the electrodes.

The results of this do-it-yourself experiment surpassed all expectations. The rats at once fell into a frenzy of self-stimulation. They pressed the pedal repeatedly, as often as 5,000 times an hour. They seemed insatiable. If allowed to, they would stimulate themselves for twenty-four hours at a stretch, stopping for neither food nor rest, until they dropped from exhaustion – and then return for another orgy a few minutes later. They would do almost anything to get a chance at the pedal: learn to run mazes rapidly and without error, remember their way the next day, and even cross electrified grids which produced shocks so painful that they had stopped starving rats from reaching food.

Over the next decade, Dr Olds diligently mapped out the rewarding areas in rats' brains. He found a 'river of reward': the medial forebrain bundle of the hypothalamus, a pathway leading from the hypothalamus to olfactory systems in the cortex. This river was dotted with 'islands' of drive. And once they were satisfied, all these drives – whether hunger, sex or thirst – seemed to produce similar feelings of reward. The stimulation apparently tapped the brain's normal mechanism for positive reinforcement, the system through which all creatures learn to do what is good for them.

At first Dr Olds held a highly optimistic view of the proportion of rewarding areas in the brain. 'I used to say that 35 per cent of the emotion-producing areas were rewarding,' Dr Olds recalled, 'that 5 per cent were punishing, and 60 per cent neutral. But that was at a time when our definitions were less adequate than today.' This optimistic view failed to hold up when it was discovered that in some cases a rat would work just as hard to stop brain stimulation as it had worked to start it. 'So there you see the animal turn it on, and you say, he loves it!' Dr Olds said. 'But then you change the conditions, you see him turn it off, and you say, he hates it! Actually it's stimulating both systems. He loves it, but he can't stand it – it's that kind of a mixed thing. This altered our map considerably.'

It stands to reason that the systems for negative and positive reinforcement should be right next to one another, Dr Olds explains, since both are involved in the animal's voluntary behaviour. He now believes that the purely positive areas in the brain – those where the rat will turn on stimulation but never work to turn it off – take up only 1 to 9 per cent of the total brain area that produces emotion. Roughly the same amount of brain matter is purely punishing. And an extraordinarily large proportion – close to half of the emotion-producing areas – gives mixed results.

Of course the situation may be quite different in different species. Cats, for example, have much more of their brain devoted to pure punishment than to pure pleasure – which may explain their generally melancholy disposition. This makes rats seem relatively well off, since they have an equal chance at either emotion. To date, nobody has drawn an atlas of the brain areas that produce exclusive pleasure or punishment in man. Dr H. J. Campbell, a physiologist at the Institute of Psychiatry in London, believes that human beings have a unique ability to activate their pleasure areas through *thinking*, as well as through sensory activity. Only human beings can have fun with mathematics, crossword puzzles or anticipation, he writes, and in his opinion, 'It is pleasure-by-thinking that separates humans from lower animals.' Unfortunately, anticipation and thinking are just as likely to produce a very human kind of pain.

Sensory pleasure has its limits. It is always conditional: food gives pleasure only if the animal is hungry, water only if the animal is thirsty, sex only if the animal has a high hormone level (though Dr Olds points out that sex powers itself to a larger degree than some other drives, and has 'fewer aversive conditions at the boundaries'). A child who loves chocolate will gorge himself only up to a certain point. But if the chocolate did not fill his stomach, he might go on eating it forever, just as a thirsty animal will continually lick at a column of air that is cold and feels wet, even though it does not satisfy its thirst. If one could stimulate the child's brain, instead of putting the chocolate in his mouth, perhaps one might have a force as irresistible as the Pied Piper's.

The brains of all animals, from fish to dolphins and primates, enclose some pleasure mechanism of this kind, where stimulation seems to act as the supreme reward. Not surprisingly, psychologists have been quick to take advantage of it. For over a decade, stimulation in the pleasure areas has been a standard operating procedure in many laboratories where animals are trained to learn certain skills. Thousands of creatures of all sizes and shapes now wear crowns of electrodes that reach down to their hypothalamus. When the stimulation is linked to a computer, as in the case of Paddy, brain rewards produce particularly quick results, and they are clearly preferable to brain pain.

Then what about using them in human beings? At this question, Dr Olds looked unhappy. 'I don't expect any wide-spread use of this methodology in humans,' he began. 'It's ex-tremely gross, in the sense that we have no idea what we are really doing when we put a probe in the brain. We know that most of the places that we localize are not the important centres. *Actually there are no brain centres.* There is a bundle of fibres running through this region carrying all of the possible emotional messages of this animal. It's as if we had tapped into a trunk line from Chicago to New York. When we turn on the current we just "say" everything at once. Almost every stimu-lated brain effect ever discovered happens in the same area. This is always the hypothalamus and almost always in its lateral part. This is the whole bundle of the brain's motivational and autonomic fibres brought through one small tube. Well, the so-called centres are just chance conglomerations of fibres, of stems, which carry the main emotional outflow of the brain past a certain point. It's not a very good way to do anything specific.'

Although he agreed to the word 'pleasure' when *Scientific American* printed an article about his work in 1956, Dr Olds, a professor of behavioural biology at the California Institute of Technology and a scientist's scientist, known for his meticulous research, is no longer so sure that pleasure was always involved. Often it was, but in some cases the brain stimulation just caused a compulsion to come back for more. 'You might call these compulsive behaviour centres,' he said. 'Others might have some relation to itching. Maybe the brain probe causes the subject to itch and brain stimulation is the only way he can scratch it.' No one yet knows where any of these motivational fibres originate, though the bundle is the only place where there are enough of them to get any effect at all. For this reason, he has now abandoned brain stimulation as a behaviour-shaping technique. Instead, he has gone back to food rewards. He believes they are more dependable.

The reports of human patients who have had electrodes implanted in their brains have not made the picture any clearer. At the Tulane University School of Medicine in New Orleans, Dr Robert Heath, one of the most daring psychiatrists in the United States, has inserted electrodes into the brains of scores of schizophrenics and other patients 'for the relief of intractable pain – emotional or physical', as he puts it. For this he is hated by Freudians, who look upon him as a sort of devil, and admired – with reservations – by some physicians who take a more biological approach to mental illness. He believes that schizophrenics cannot experience pleasure in the same way as other people because of a defect in the septal region of their brains, a part of the limbic system. He treats them with electric stimulation which, he claims, produces the pleasure they have always missed. Some of his patients have been equipped with control boxes that allow them to stimulate their own pleasure centres at will. And some have reported feelings that range from mild euphoria to something 'better than sex'. When the electrodes were placed in areas that produced the most intense self-stimulation, however, the patients seemed unable to explain their actions. If asked why they stimulated themselves, they might say, 'Because Dr Heath will give me more passes to go home if I do,' or name some other thing they remembered doing on purpose. Another odd trait of these patients was that in several cases they didn't stop pushing the lever after the electricity was turned off. They went right on, repetitively, as if they didn't know the difference.

'You can't know the human brain as well as an animal brain,' Dr Olds points out. 'You can slice animal brains literally

55

by the thousands and mark your target every time you aim at something, then see how you did. Then you aim again and slice, and pretty soon you learn by that kind of marking your target where you're going. Now, very few people sacrifice their human subjects [he smiles wryly], therefore no one ever learns where he is going in the human brain. One surgeon, Dr Vernon Mark of Boston, did try to simulate this technique,' said Dr Olds. 'What Dr Mark did was get himself a couple of hundred cadavers and implant in them, and then slice the brains. So he's to be praised for having created, for himself and his group at least, human stereotactic procedure.' Dr Mark's work, with Dr Frank Ervin, in stimulating the brains of cancer patients to relieve them of pain sounds to Dr Olds 'like something I might approve of – one of the few possible uses of this technique'. However, any invasion of the brain involves real risks, particularly the danger that it may build up scar tissue, which could provoke epileptic seizures. Dr Olds warns that implanted electrodes always create as many troubles as they cure, though in the process one learns a little more about the brain.

Now in his fifties and as conservative in appearance as he is cautious in his thinking, Dr Olds has become very concerned about the possible consequences of recent brain research. In 1971, when I asked him about the dangers that might be posed by electrical stimulation of the brain, he scoffed at them. 'Wild therapeutic procedures have a relatively small and self-restricting vogue,' he said, 'and then they eventually disappear. Society gets rid of them. Most of the work that is being done with probes implanted in human brains will fall into that category. Occasionally people come along and say how terrible, everyone will have his brain implanted. You know, most people don't even let themselves be injected intraperitoneally, because it looks like being stabbed in the stomach. Do you think they're going to bow their heads down and say, "Please drill a hole in my top"? It's really kind of foolish.'

Today he is no longer in a joking mood. He emphasizes that a brain stimulus is a pathology. The electrode itself is unnatural, and the stimulation even more so. Together they create a sort of disease, 'somewhat like knocking a man out with a sledge-hammer and then asking what colour stars he sees'. No brain stimulation that we know how to provide would be likely to pro-duce more than something like the 'aura' that precedes an epilep-tic fit. A person pursuing a 'brain reward' might well end up by begging a doctor for a cure: he might hate the stimulus but be unable to stop himself. 'We know only where a mixed bag of emotional fibres happens to be passing, where we can induce a rather sickly pathological condition,' Dr Olds concluded.

If we want to tap into any of the fibres that specifically pro-duce pleasure, we will have to develop far more sophisticated ways of getting to them. We not only need better electrodes, we need a much better idea of where to put them.

In a way, this is quite reassuring. On the other hand, if we do learn more about these fibres, we may eventually be able to put them to good use in various kinds of therapy. In recent years, there has been mounting evidence that people can be trained to control their own heart rate, blood pressure and other supposedly involuntary functions, with help from a computer. If such control can be achieved at all, the most direct route for the computer's feedback is directly to the brain. The computer could screen the information from a man's heart, for instance, and every time his heart rate changed in the appropriate direc-tion, order instant pleasure in the man's brain. 'I like the idea,' says Dr Olds, 'even though I can't really believe it. You see, if you could feed back certain cardiac responses to brain stimula-tion, you might cause long-lasting changes in heart rate and thus resolve illnesses that have a psychosomatic origin. The whole circle might be totally unconscious.' The heart rate would be modified by these rewards, without the patient consciously deciding what to do.

As Dr Delgado's experiment with Paddy showed, remote con-trol of this sort is now possible, and it is a superb training device. With a brain implant to give him imperceptible jolts every time his heart rate was lowered, a cardiac patient might calm himself during stressful situations until his heart reached a normal level – at which point, like a good thermostat, the computer would order the stimulation to stop. All these events might remain inaccessible to his cortex. The patient would then find various rationalizations for his good temper, from the kindness of the people around him to the pleasantness of the weather.

The micro-miniaturization of electronic equipment is proceeding at such a fast pace that small, reliable, efficient brain implants may be expected within a decade. Engineers are not lacking in ideas on how to power them internally. To do away with batteries (and the need to replace or recharge them), they want a permanent source of energy. What could be more convenient than to harness the energy produced by the body itself? Some researchers hope to convert the oxygen contained in the body into a source of power. By inserting two electrodes into the skeletal muscle of animals, for instance – one of platinum, to reduce oxygen and release electrons, the other of aluminium, to increase oxidation and take up electrons – experimenters have already succeeded in obtaining 100 microwatts of power at about one volt. Others are betting on the energy released by the rhythmic expansion and contraction of blood vessels during circulation. And if all else fails, they could embed a tiny source of atomic energy in the brain, right along with the mechanism it would fuel.

Bridging the span between a man's brain and the computer would be even less of a problem. Even today, epileptic patients' EEGs can be transmitted accurately, via ordinary telephone lines, to specialists 2,000 miles away, and astronauts' brain waves can be recorded in flight, then telemetered back to earth with the greatest of ease. In brain research, as in jet travel, distance has become nearly meaningless.

The closer we come to such remote control of the brain, however, the more logical Delgado's next plan appears. This would elminate the problem of distance, but in an entirely different manner. Delgado would simply put everything inside the patient – not just the stimoceiver or dialytrode and its source of power, but the computer as well. Naturally he would need a very tiny, miniaturized computer, smaller than anything available today, but he is confident that it can be built. 'Then the whole electronics would be inside the body,' he exclaimed. 'No radio link would be necessary. The process would be going on in a closed circuit, totally inside the subject.'

The implants, whether electrical or chemical, would be sealed into the brain for good, their action directed by the implanted computer. If the computer's programme needed to be changed, one could still have access to it from outside, just as one changes T V channels by remote control.

A man with such an implant would feel a 'compulsion' to behave along the lines planned for him. For the rest of his life, the computer would shape him, sending periodic jolts of pain or pleasure directly to his brain – and neither he nor anyone around him would know it.

The next decade may see a growing tug of war between those who are seduced by such technology and scientists who realize that they still know far too little about what really happens when one invades the human brain.

4 Controlling one's own brain waves: the beautiful world of bio-feedback

At the opposite extreme from the efforts to manipulate the brains of others, a movement to teach people how to control their own brains has been gathering speed in recent years. Some of the nation's most imaginative researchers are now involved in it, as well as thousands of students, volunteers and camp followers of all kinds. Together they are soaring off into a beautiful world where everything seems possible – the world of bio-feedback.

It is not necessary to drill a hole in the skull to control the brain, they say. Nor is it necessary to take drugs. All one needs is concentration, coupled with precise information on what's going on in one's brain *at the time it occurs*. Then, with training, one can achieve the kind of self-control that people have always dreamed of but seldom attained. One can become oblivious to pain, exceptionally alert, or fall into a creative reverie, at will.

Of course yogis and Zen masters have known such skills for years, but they learn them the hard way, through a lifetime of meditation and study. In the West we want speed as well as hard evidence. Today, both have become available through bio-feedback, a technique that depends on electronic gadgets which measure and amplify physiological changes so small that until recently they were almost totally ignored.

By now hundreds of volunteers have learned to produce small changes in their blood pressure, lower their heart rates, alter their brain rhythms or stop the activity of a single cell in their spinal cord – functions previously believed to be involuntary, or beyond human control.

They have done all this without drugs, and without black magic. For bio-feedback simply extends normal ways of learning. Everything we learn depends on some sort of feedback – from eyes, ears, hands, feet, other people or other sources – that shows us whether we are succeeding or failing in what we are trying to do. But under normal circumstances, we are limited in the kind of feedback we can get from our body. We don't have words to say what's going on inside us. Very often we can't even identify it. Small increases or decreases in blood pressure remain hidden from consciousness. So do changes in the rhythm of our brain waves. With the aid of sensitive bio-feedback equipment, however, such internal fluctuations can be measured, displayed and evaluated instantly to tell the learner whether he is improving.

It's somewhat like helping a blindfolded man learn to type. He could never make any progress if he didn't know what letters he was producing. But if someone told him the name of each key as he struck it, he could begin to type certain letters at will. With time and practice, he could even learn to type rapidly, until at last his fingers would seem to do their work by themselves. Suppose the person who named these keys also handed the man a raisin as a reward for each letter he typed correctly. This would be called operant conditioning – the kind of training, systematized by B. F. Skinner, in which rewards (or positive reinforcements) are used to shape behaviour. If the man had strong reasons of his own for wanting to type, however, simply *knowing* that he had struck the right key would be its own reward.

'You *must* care,' said Dr Neal Miller of Rockefeller University, 'otherwise the results cannot be rewarding.' In bio-feedback rapid signals such as a flash of light or a beep show the volunteer that he is doing well. While taking part in an experiment at Harvard Medical School, I was amazed at how much I cared. Sitting alone in a dimly lit, soundproofed room, with no distractions and nothing to do but focus on the beep, I began to feel elated every time I heard it. I didn't know what the experimenters had decided to reward (it turned out to be lower blood pressure, combined with a lower heart rate), nor what I was doing to earn it, but every time the beep went on it was like hitting the jackpot. What surprised me most, however, was the speed with which everything took place. The beeps sometimes followed each other incredibly rapidly – up to thirty-two times a minute. (At other times, of course, there were long, dull periods without any evidence of success.) As the psychophysiologist Bernard Tursky explained, the signals had to be almost instantaneous so as to reward the appropriate heartbeat and allow me to control the next one, which came less than a second later. The speed at which the body works is the strength of biofeedback. Just because of the short time-lapse between heartbeats, one can learn very rapidly, through much trial and error, while the clock hand barely moves.

Bio-feedback, then, requires lightning-swift measurements, rapid calculations of whether each change is a step forwards or backwards and instant displays. It is a child of the computer age. But it might never have developed without the persistence and wide influence of Dr Miller, a psychologist, who maintained for years that the body's internal functions could be brought under voluntary control, even though the textbooks said this was impossible.

Dr Miller, who had won fame for his book *Social Learning and Imitation*, written with John Dollard in 1941, stood nearly alone in his belief that, through practice, one could learn to control the internal organs and glands, just as one controls the skeletal muscles (arms, legs and other visible parts). The skeletal muscles are triggered off by the motor area of the cortex, through nerves running down the centre of the spine. Internal responses are regulated by the 'emotional' areas of the brain – the limbic system, and particularly the hypothalamus – through two chains of nerve fibres travelling down the sides of the spinal cord. Ever since Plato, people have considered these internal functions to be somehow inferior. The nervous system that controls them was supposedly involuntary and independent – hence its name, the autonomic nervous system. Most psychologists believed that it could be conditioned in the classical way, using Pavlov's methods, but could not be taught through trial and error. Pavlov's dog salivated naturally at the sight of food. When a bell consistently preceded the food, the dog learned to associate the two, and eventually began to salivate at the sound of the bell, even when no food was presented. However, it could not be expected to learn any response other than salivation. Skinner taught pigeons skills that no pigeon had ever had before – for example, how to play ping-pong – through a step-by-step reinforcement of some of the movements they produced by trial and error. Such methods were reserved for the skeletal muscles, however. In the traditional view, the autonomic nervous system was too 'stupid' to learn by operant conditioning.

The shortcomings of the autonomic nervous system seemed so obvious that Dr Miller had a terrible time convincing any students to work on what later became bio-feedback. Even the paid assistants whom he assigned to the project did it half-heartedly, believing it was a waste of time. Finally, a young man, Jay Trowill, volunteered to run some experiments. He faced an immense technical problem: proving that any change in a rat's heart rate resulted from direct control over the heart itself, and not from some other muscular exertion to speed up the heart, or relaxation to slow it down. It was extremely difficult to prevent such 'cheating'. After a series of discouraging attempts Trowill paralysed his rats with curare, the substance that South American Indians use in poison arrows. This stopped them from using any skeletal muscles at all. Since curare does not affect the internal organs, however, the rats could still use their heart muscles. They lay limp and inert on the experimenters' table, unable to move their lungs, their little pointed noses and mouths inserted into tiny face masks (made from toy balloons) which led to respirators that maintained their breathing. In this totally helpless condition, the rats were required to control their heart rates. Of course none of the ordinary rewards such as food or

water held much appeal for them. So the experimenters implanted electrodes into the rats' brains and stimulated their
pleasure centres every time their heart rates changed in the
desired direction. Some rats were rewarded for speeding up their
heart, and others were rewarded for slowing it down. By 1966,
after three years of painstaking work, Trowill had unequivocal
proof that rats could achieve direct control over their heart rates,
without any assistance from their skeletal muscles.

As soon as the rats learned to produce small increases or
decreases in heart rate, Dr Miller and Leo DiCara, his principal
associate, increased their demands—from then on, the rewards
came only for bigger and bigger changes. By 'shaping' the rats'
heart rates in this way, they produced changes of roughly 20 per
cent in either direction, after only ninety minutes of training –
an almost unbelievable speed.

Clearly, the mechanism for self-control of the internal organs
was there. Not only was it there, it was also surprisingly precise.
Drs Miller and DiCara pride themselves on having trained some
rats to perform a yoga-like trick: dilating the blood vessels in
one ear more than those in the other, a sophistication which Dr
Miller finds 'eerie'.

These results opened up all parts of the nervous system, the
internal organs and the glands to highly specific forms of training. None of these was 'beyond voluntary control' any more.
'There is only one kind of learning,' Dr Miller declared happily.
'We are now forced into a radical reorientation of thinking about
functions ordinarily concealed inside the body.'

Soon a number of patients whose hearts skipped a beat
succeeded in training their hearts to beat in a normal manner
through bio-feedback – at least in the laboratory. Others, who
suffered from hypertension, learned to lower their blood pressure, though the changes were too small to be very useful.
Migraine patients cured themselves of headaches by increasing
the blood flow in their hands, which relieved their heads. These
changes were not as dramatic as those in animals, nor did the
people involved learn as rapidly, probably because the training

conditions could not be controlled as carefully – nobody wants to be paralysed by curare, even though this seems to clear the decks for learning and to prevent such errors as using the skeletal muscles to fake progress. (Rats that have not been treated with curare also learn more slowly.) Much work remains to be done before it can be used as effective therapy. Nevertheless, there is growing evidence of success with bio-feedback, especially in the control of the brain.

Dr Miller and his group had noticed something strange about the rats in their heart experiment: those that had been trained to speed up their hearts seemed more 'emotional' – they squealed, squirmed and defecated more – than those that had been trained to make their heart rates go down. Their brains also contained more of certain neurotransmitters, which meant that their central nervous systems had become more excitable. Evidently the change in their heart rate had triggered off changes in their brain chemistry as well as their behaviour.

The next step was to try to train the brain directly. This time cats were the subject – they were wide-awake, not treated with curare, and could move freely despite the long wires connecting their heads to lab instruments. The wires led to electrodes implanted in their brains' pleasure centres. A graduate student, Alfredo Carmona, stimulated some cats in these pleasure centres every time they lowered the voltage of their brain waves, and others whenever they raised it. Before long, he had two different kinds of cats on his hands. The group that had been rewarded for high-voltage, low-frequency brain waves 'sat like sphinxes, staring out into space', Dr Miller recalled. The other cats, which had learned to produce low-voltage, faster waves paced about restlessly, sniffing and looking around. To make sure that this was happening through direct control of the brain, and not through eye movements or some other activity of the skeletal muscles, Carmona repeated the experiment with rats treated with curare and proved that they could change the rhythm of their brain waves at will.

Could human beings learn as well? 'I believe that men are

as clever as rats,' said Dr Miller. 'However, we may not yet be as clever at training them.'

Very fittingly, the first person to offer evidence of Zen-like control over the brain through bio-feedback was a serene psychologist of Japanese descent, Dr Joe Kamiya, of the Langley-Porter Neuropsychiatric Institute in San Francisco, whose early experiments antedated the Rockefeller work. Dr Kamiya had come to the problem from quite a different angle. He had long been interested in states of consciousness – the inner states that change so radically during dreams, under drugs and at other times. However, his training as a behaviourist made such vague concepts as 'mind' or 'consciousness' taboo as subjects for research. Behaviourists were supposed to study only what could be measured – specific stimuli and responses. So, while doing conventional research on E E G changes during sleep and dreams in Chicago in 1958, Dr Kamiya 'bootlegged' some work on the E E Gs of people who were wide-awake. He wanted to see whether he could train them to recognize the comings and goings of various rhythms in their brains, starting with the most prominent rhythm of all, the alpha rhythm, which Berger had discovered in 1924. He pasted electrodes on their scalp, watched the pattern of their brain waves on an E E G, and rang a bell sometimes when the alpha rhythm was present, sometimes when it was absent, asking the volunteers to guess which state they were in. Every time he rang the bell they had to reply, and each time he told them whether they were right or wrong. During the first hour they usually guessed right only half the time, which suggests that nothing more than chance was operating. But by the second hour of training they could guess right 60 per cent of the time, and by the third hour they were right 75 to 80 per cent of the time and after a while some of the volunteers could actually guess right every single time – as often as 400 times in a row!

'The subject had learned to read his own brain, or his mind,' Dr Kamiya announced. 'He had become aware of an internal state.'

Even more exciting was something Dr Kamiya discovered by accident: having learned to recognize his alpha waves, one of the volunteers also knew how to turn them on or off at will. And when Dr Kamiya tested the others, he found that all his subjects were able to do so, at least to some extent.

Now that was a really extraordinary development, and when Dr Kamiya moved to California he set out at once to see whether people could be trained to control their brain waves without first going through the discrimination phase. He found that they could. The ten volunteers in his experiment had no previous preparation. They simply sat in dark, soundproof rooms, with electrodes on their heads, and tried to keep a tone sounding. They were told that the tone was turned on by their brain waves when they were in certain mental states. After a while they were told to try to keep the tone *off* as much as possible. At the end of forty reversals, eight out of the ten could control the tone. When asked to turn it on, they had alpha waves 55 per cent of the time, and when asked to turn it off their production of alpha dropped down to 17 per cent.

However, they didn't quite know how they did it. They knew only that it couldn't be forced. The more they tried to produce alpha, especially at the beginning, the less they had. They would try all kinds of tricks: mental arithmetic, thinking sexy thoughts, listening to their breathing, or focusing on the back of their head, all to no avail. Then they would give up – and suddenly improve. 'Gradually they'd sift out *the* crucial mental state from what's irrelevant,' Dr Kamiya said. It usually took at least four or five sessions to gain any real control. Once they had achieved good control, however, they retained this skill for weeks or months. Of the hundreds of volunteers he has trained so far, nearly all preferred alpha to the non-alpha state.

What's so good about being in alpha? I asked Dr Kamiya. 'Here are the words that subjects use to describe it,' he replied. 'Calm; alert; relaxed; open to experiences of all kinds; pleasant, in the sense that to be serene is pleasant, as opposed to the hassle of American life. It's akin to the good feeling that comes from taking a massage or sauna bath – a relaxed, put-together sort of feeling. It's receptive, as opposed to a getting, forcing frame of mind. You have to let it occur spontaneously, then be happy you have it.'

The alpha state itself is probably not creative, he explained. 'But a poet told me that just before he's ready to write a good poem, he's in a state that seems very similar to high alpha. You see, alpha is a state of attention directed towards letting things happen.' How can it be a state of attention, if you can't focus your attention on anything in particular? I asked. 'That's one of the most peculiar things about it,' said Dr Kamiya. 'It's probably best described as a shift in the focus of attention. You can't let yourself get drowsy, as this would take you out of alpha. You remain alert, expanding your focus of attention in all directions.'

Brain waves in the alpha range – a frequency of 8 to 13 cycles per second – may represent the brain's way of idling between states of high mental activity and sleep. Some people, especially those who are introspective and intuitive, normally produce large quantities of alpha, while others produce very little. The reasons for this difference are unknown. Nor is it known which of these groups benefits more from training, though all kinds of people can learn to increase their output.

When Dr Kamiya's subjects told him they felt calm and tranquil in alpha, he realized at once that this sounded like a Zen state. But he didn't like the idea. Dr Kamiya was still a proper behaviourist, and he hadn't planned to dabble in meditation; he thought he was conditioning alpha. The temptation was too strong, however, and finally he hooked up some experienced Zen meditators to his E E G feedback system, just to see how they would do. When they learned to control their alpha waves much more rapidly than other people, he was forced to take notice.

'And so we found ourselves at the back door of a centuries-old tradition that we, in the West, have very little understanding of,' he said. 'Right now in the U.S., a growing number of people, especially college students, are interested in meditation. Many of them seem to have cultivated their interest through drugs such as L S D. But I don't think it's transitory – some interest in Eastern meditation practices will be here in our culture to stay.'

In Sanskrit there are twenty different names for varying states of 'consciousness' or 'mind' – yet we are limited to these two words. If Dr Kamiya's subjects find it so difficult to give satisfactory verbal descriptions of their experiences while turning on alpha, it may be partly a language problem. However, he believes it really reflects the fact that 'we have not been trained to name various physiological states. As children we have never been spanked or rewarded for them. Nor do we sit around the living room talking about how much alpha we've had.'

He hopes that a 'vocabulary of moods' will soon be developed, a vocabulary much more precise than the words available to poets today. If you were a Martian and wanted to find out the earthlings' dimensions of taste, he notes, you could start out with sweet, sour, salty and bitter, since all tastes are combinations thereof. But how would you begin to understand human moods and feelings? What are their basic dimensions? His long-range goal is to develop co-ordinates for the various qualities of experience associated with brain-wave changes. Then one could describe a melancholy mood, for instance, as a specific point on this map of consciousness. Dr Kamiya is no longer an orthodox behaviourist, but he still believes in precise techniques. 'We must be able to index our experience,' he said.

Dr Kamiya's vision of the future is one of benign, even beneficent technology. He visualizes a person of the twenty-first century sitting in an armchair, with electrodes pasted to his head and connected to a musical instrument. Each musical tone would be controlled by certain brain-wave dimensions. No muscular participation would be required. The person would be expected only to sit back and listen to his moods. 'He would lead his own orchestra, so to speak. He would feel himself,' says Dr Kamiya. In a way, it would be idiosyncratic music. But since all human beings are wired up in basically the same fashion, the tonal patterns associated with different moods might be pretty much alike for different persons. Others might then be invited to listen in.

'Two lovers facing each other and a panel of lights or tones could play interesting games, or communicate in this complex way,' Dr Kamiya suggests. 'They would be freed of the difficulties people so often have when they try to express their emotions in words. They could flirt through their brain waves.'

Another Kamiya vision, which he finds less attractive, involves children with little light bulbs on top of their heads. Most teachers long for a way to know whether their pupils are really paying attention or just daydreaming, he notes. Individual alpha-sensors might be the answer to their prayers. If each child had one, connected to a light bulb on top of his head, his light would shine whenever he was in alpha. This would warn his teacher that he wasn't concentrating. On the other hand, if few of the children's lights were on in a classroom, the teacher would know they were all working hard – unless, of course, they were drowsy or asleep, which also stops the alpha rhythm.

Turning this around, Dr Kamiya foresees a new kind of sensitivity training in which children would become aware of the goings-on inside their bodies and their minds and, eventually, learn to control them. 'Just as children are sometimes blindfolded and asked to name the objects they touch, to give them experience in sensing the outside world, they might be attached to feedback machines to learn about their inside world,' he said. 'They might learn that when they have certain emotions, their palms sweat, or that when they're excited, their hearts beat faster. I'll bet a lot of kids, and certainly adults, don't know when they're angry. I think it's good for a child to know if he's angry, or happy, or anxious, to explore himself in different states of mind.' After such training, even young children should be able to talk fluently about the 'feel' of certain brain waves, or of changes in blood pressure. They should know how to deploy their attention with unusual efficiency. Perhaps they would also learn to produce more alpha, which should at least help them to relax.

Dr Kamiya himself doesn't do 'any of the meditation things'. He hasn't even sat much in his lab practising alpha rhythms – he's far too busy. Perhaps a man who can stop in the middle of a business meeting to go out and admire the cherry blossoms before the sun sets, as he did in Washington recently, doesn't really need more alpha. Nevertheless, a cult has grown around his experiments, and he is deluged by letters and phone calls from people all over the country who beg him to let them serve as subjects so that they can get an 'alpha high'.

The people who do become his subjects soon develop a jargon of their own, comparing their different brain-wave experiences as they might compare the pleasures of drugs or sex. They like being in alpha. In many cases, it comes to replace marijuana or LSD.

Other eager students line up by the hundreds at the labs of the other pioneers in this field, especially that of Dr Barbara Brown, of the Veterans Administration hospital in Sepulveda, California, and that of Dr Lester Fehmi, of the Medical Center at Princeton, New Jersey. By now more than 100 different research labs are working on brain-wave training, and the number seems to double every year.

But as fast as the legitimate research grows, the quacks proliferate even faster. They moved in as soon as alpha training hit the nation's campuses, and publicity in the mass-circulation magazines helped them along. California attracts the most vociferous hawkers, who promise people anything – weight loss, the man or woman of their choice, intuition – through expensive alpha-training.

There is also a nationwide chain of 'Silva Mind Control' courses, which offer to teach 'the new science of Alphagenics', or the control of brain waves, at $200 a time – but does not even use an EEG machine! Special Seminars in Silva Mind Control have been advertised in leading newspapers, luring thousands of people to a sales talk (which itself costs $5 per person to hear) during which they are told that Mind Control accelerates healing, controls pain, produces more 'energy-vitality', success and intuition, leads to a higher 'IQ factor', improves sleep, brings more friends and so on. Claiming over 10,000 graduates from coast to coast, the ads describe Silva as a parapsychologist from the Institute of Psychorientology (whatever that is) in Laredo, Texas. He is said to have developed clairvoyance to such a degree that one of his students, an eight-year-old girl, could close her eyes and not only describe where one should drill for oil, but also what quality that oil would be.

Perhaps one can't really blame the Mind Control people for dispensing with alpha-feedback machines, considering the bugs in all but the most expensive models. Several manufacturers are now developing supposedly reliable bio-feedback trainers of various kinds, which should soon be available for less than $200 each. But the alpha trainers that one can buy for home practice at present either don't work or pick up too much interference from household current, eyeblinks and other artifacts to be of any use. When I tried one recently – on my husband, who volunteered to go first – we had a maddening time trying to interpret the machine's beeps and wheezes, which were supposed to represent alpha but came on only when the electrodes were jiggled accidentally, or when they were not attached to his scalp at all. Meanwhile, our nine-year-old son walked in and yelped with joy to see his father wearing an Indian-style strap around his forehead, with wires dangling from his head. He rushed upstairs to round up his older brother and a friend and show them the sight, despite our pleas that 'the subject must not be disturbed . . .' It turned out later that the machine was out of order, as often happens. It seems that our experience was not unique. Many researchers are hampered in their experiments because they have no equipment to give their trainees for home use.

There are definite limits, then, to alpha training at home. Yet it has limits even in a research lab, with the best of equipment. In a speech before the Massachusetts Psychological

Association in May 1971, Dr Thomas Mulholland, chairman of the recently formed Bio-Feedback Research Society, threw some cold water on what he called 'the alpha cult'. There is no evidence that having lots of alpha rhythms is associated with any special mental powers, he declared. There is no evidence that it brings relief from physical or mental disease. It is *not* instant yoga. Alpha is the commonest phenomenon in the EEG: if you close your eyes, you usually get a burst of alpha, and most of us slip in and out of alpha several times a minute. Ordinary people with no insight into meditation will show large quantities of alpha. Children will, too. Millions of people have lots of alpha – but not many people meditate under those circumstances, or develop insights into themselves. Dr Mulholland suggested that the state of quiet in which people must remain during alpha training might be the real cause of most of its so-called benefits.

'By taking time out to be relaxed yet awake for an hour in a quiet place, people are finding out that they have thoughts,' he said acidly. 'For some, this experience assumes the status of a major insight.' The content of their thoughts and the quality of their moods during that time are not specific to alpha, however. Rather, they depend on the person's expectations or fears. In some cases,' he said, 'the tone (which indicates alpha) becomes so valued that hearing it makes them feel successful, comfortable and relaxed, while not hearing it brings expressions of failure, discontent and tension, even when the alpha occurrence is about the same.'

He did concede that if a person has alpha, he must be relaxed. Hence, training in alpha could be useful for those who are normally too tense, though of course there are many other ways of relaxing as well. In Dr Mulholland's own lab, subjects are taught not how to increase their production of alpha, but how to suppress it, to see whether this will lead to higher levels of attention.

Between this negative position and the exaggerated claims of the alpha charlatans lie two facts: (1) Some people can learn

73

to control their own brain waves with bio-feedback, at least to some extent; and (2) there is far more to brain rhythms than alpha – and even alpha consists of several slightly different rhythms.

Most of the researchers who have worked with alpha feedback have reported striking success. Barbara Brown writes that in her California laboratory 'the average subject had more than doubled the amount of alpha in his E E G by the end of the first practice session, and tripled the amount in the third practice session. The increase in abundance of alpha occurred with the eyes open [this is supposedly much more difficult, since closing one's eyes almost automatically produces alpha] and while the subject was trying to keep the light on [her feedback signal was a blue light, rather than a beep].' By the third practice session, their production of alpha reached a maximum of 60 per cent of all E E G activity – as much as or more than the average person shows when he has his eyes closed and is very relaxed. She adds that her trained subjects achieved such control that eventually they were able to do without E E G feedback. They simply turned alpha on or off at will.

In her next experiment, she used lights of three different colours to represent three different kinds of waves: alpha, beta and theta. Our understanding of these basic brain rhythms is still so primitive that Dr Brown simply tried to find out what sort of feelings or moods are related to each one. Beta waves (14 to 30 cycles per second) are faster and smaller than alpha (8 to 13 cycles per second). Theta waves (4 to 7 cycles per second) run slower and bigger than alpha. And the slowest waves of all, delta (which she did not include in the experiment), vary between .5 and 3.5 cycles per second, a rhythm dominant in sleep, in infancy and in brain disease.

After watching the coloured lights change – a reflection of the change in their brain waves – Dr Brown's twenty-six subjects wrote down what they had felt during each colour. The alpha state was generally experienced as pleasant and tranquil. During the faster beta state, fourteen persons reported feeling worry, anger, fear, frustration or excitement. Theta, the rarest state, did not stand out too clearly in their minds, but eight persons reported that they had been busy with some sort of problem-solving. According to Dr Brown, the consistency of the comments about each state showed that people can identify different rhythms in their brain. She hopes that training in the theta rhythm will lead to 'a sensational increase in the efficacy with which the mind works'.

It may turn out that the most interesting changes in consciousness come not from being in alpha more of the time, but from *changing the frequency of one's alpha waves*, or going into theta. This, too, can be learned, judging from preliminary experiments at the Menninger Foundation, the well-known psychiatric centre in Topeka, Kansas.

Some strange things have been going on in Topeka recently, and the good doctors in the clinical department, which is concerned with such practical matters as making sick people well, are watching it all with mixed feelings – from a distance. In a spanking new building surrounded by greenery, the Gardner Murphy Research Building, Dr Elmer Green, Director of the Psychophysiology Lab, is trying to train people to go into states of creative reverie. He worked on weapons development until the age of thirty-seven, but spent the next four years studying physiological psychology at the University of Chicago. There he became fascinated by the problem of how the unconscious processes in mind and body work together – how one can speed up healing, for instance, by inner control. 'Everybody knows that if you worry, you can get ulcers,' he said. 'If that's true, the opposite is also true! If there is psychosomatic illness, there is also psychosomatic health. The thing that isn't understood is how the lower brain centres control healing, how they're programmed.'

Body and mind fit together almost perfectly, so that if you disturb one, the other is also disturbed. That's why chemicals work as mood- and emotion-changers, he says. On the other hand, 'if you give people some good news, maybe a dozen

75

important physiological processes go through change. Bad news can make them faint. Both sets of changes occur just because they heard somebody say something.'

Dr Green's studies aim at finding out how a person's will enters into the picture – how it can bring about such changes in body and brain. He refers to hypnosis as a sort of shortcut, in which the subject's attention is so fixed on the hypnotist that there is less activity in the cortex (which is why subjects later report amnesia for this period), and the hypnotist can talk directly to the lower centres of the subject's brain. He has been much influenced by the work of a German doctor, Johannes Schultz, who developed a system of self-regulation called autogenic training early in this century. Despite its considerable success, autogenic training has remained almost unknown in the United States. Dr Green happened to see a British book on it while he was in Chicago in 1959, and he liked its combination of the self-control aspects of yoga with some techniques taken from medical hypnosis. 'About the time that Freud gave up hypnosis as a tool because it was undependable,' he says, 'Schultz decided that it apparently was undependable because the patient, not being in control of this situation, in one way or another sometimes resisted the doctor and prevented the entire control.' Schultz therefore put the patient in charge of the situation, in a kind of self-hypnosis coupled with graduated training exercises, and eventually taught many people to control their autonomic processes. Unfortunately, as with yoga, this took a long time to learn.

In 1964, the well-known psychologist, Gardner Murphy, invited Dr Green to come to Menninger and start a psychophysiology lab so that the Foundation's psychiatrists and psychologists could have a place to study what went on in the body during various psychological states. At the same time, Dr Murphy pointed out to Dr Green that an interesting new technique, biofeedback, had just been developed, and he suggested that Dr Green should combine it with his work on autogenic training. Dr Green was delighted. Since then he and his wife, Alyce, a psychologist, have been among the most active researchers in this field.

'Feedback is a very powerful tool,' said Dr Green, who has found it allows people to learn various forms of control much more quickly than with autogenic training alone. However, certain tasks remain extremely difficult, even with feedback, and some phrases from autogenic training seem to point people in the right direction by giving them a 'feel' of what is required.

To see how their dual system worked, I accompanied the Greens as they gave a demonstration of feedback training to a class at Unity Village, the headquarters of the Unity School of Christianity in Kansas City, Missouri. They took with them twenty-five temperature-training instruments called 'thermistors'. These were highly sensitive meters, designed at Menninger, which could detect minute changes in temperature and could be adjusted to distinguish between two parts of the body. The students, most of them middle-aged and lonely-looking, would practice with the meters for a week on their own, but during the first session the Greens wanted them to have the pure experience of relaxing, unhampered by the need to watch the needle go up or down. Therefore they worked in pairs: each student recorded his partner's progress, rather than his own, and then changed places. I mixed in with the students to try it out. When everyone was seated Mrs Green, who has worked beside her husband for years (while also raising their four children), took over the session.

The purpose of the exercise, she said, would be to make our hands get warmer and our foreheads cooler – a sign that we were relaxed. She told us to pick up the tiny thermistors, which looked like grains of pepper embedded in plastic at the tips of thin electric wires, and place one on our forehead with adhesive tape, while keeping the other stuck on the third finger of our dominant hand. 'The machine will show the change in temperature that you're accomplishing,' she said. 'But you must tell your body what to do in a way it can understand – by visualizing, imagining, feeling – that's the language of the body.'

77

In a calm, quiet tone of voice she then began to read the autogenic phrases, phrases which we were to say to ourselves as well: 'I feel quite quiet . . . I am beginning to feel quite relaxed . . . My feet feel heavy and relaxed . . . Warmth is flowing into my hands, they are warm, warm . . .' There were some noises outside the classroom, but they did not disturb us. I felt as if I had sunk into some kind of warm bath where I was getting hotter and hotter, close to sleep, vacant, aware of what was going on in the outside world but caring little about it. Time seemed to stretch out forever. When Mrs Green brought the session to an end with the words, 'I feel life and energy flowing through my legs, hips, solar plexus, chest, arms and hands, neck and head,' it was a real effort – and quite unpleasant – to come out from what had definitely been a 'different' state. I glanced at my partner, an elderly, retired businessman. He was smiling. It seems the meter had told the whole story: the temperature difference between my hands and forehead had risen from zero at the beginning of the exercise to 1 degree Fahrenheit after the fourth autogenic phrase, 2 degrees after the eighth, $2\frac{1}{2}$ after the tenth, and remained at that high level until the final phrase, when it suddenly dropped back to less than 1.

This is '*passive volition*', Dr Green explained to the class later. 'You tell the body what you want, and you let the body take over.' Blood-flow to the hands is a good tool to work with because it indicates so clearly whether the autonomic nervous system is relaxed, he said. The autonomic nervous system is a dual mechanism, consisting of the parasympathetic system, which slows down the body, preparing it for relaxation and rest, and the sympathetic system, which prepares it for fight or flight. Generally these two systems put limits on one another. But the blood-flow to the hands is controlled only by the sympathetic system, which responds to anxiety – this is why anxiety produces such cold hands. Warming the hands thus cuts down the outflow of the system that is connected with tension, and 'if you can warm up your hands, you *have* to relax the autonomic nervous system'.

It is quite an easy trick to learn. The autogenic phrases are used only at the beginning of training. The feedback meter is used for a somewhat longer time, but after a while people can even dispense with that and raise the temperature of their hands by sheer concentration. Such control is particularly useful for people who suffer from migraine or tension headaches. The Greens value it as a sort of setting-up exercise to show new subjects how easy it is to produce physical changes through the mind, and also to prepare their autonomic nervous system, which must be relaxed before they can 'go down the well' to the deeper, more internalized state the Greens call 'reverie'.

'Going down the well' of one's consciousness usually means lowering the frequency of one's brain waves, the Greens have found. In their lab, subjects reported the most interesting, dream-like images at the time that their alpha waves decreased in frequency from 10 to 8 cycles per second, or from 8 to the slower theta rhythms.

'If you want to have a creative solution to a problem you're stuck on, or a creative idea, how do you programme yourself?' asks Dr Green. He points out that people often get their most unusual ideas when they're not actively thinking about the subject. The ideas 'just sort of come in, full-blown. Quite a few people have learned to lie down and go into a reverie, or a dream-like state, for this purpose.'

Since deep reverie is usually associated with low-alpha or theta rhythms, it might be possible, through feedback, to train people to become more creative, more in tune with their unconscious, by training them to produce more theta. This is the goal of the Greens' present experiments. Having done pilot work on themselves and a group of friends (and developed, at last, enough reliable portable E E G feedback machines to allow feedback practice outside their laboratory), they are launching an ambitious programme of alpha and theta training for college students. At Washburn University, in Topeka, three machines have been placed in small rooms. A group of students practises with these machines one hour a day, every day, between weekly sessions at the Menninger lab, keeping a diary of their experiences. The images that one has during theta are usually too fleeting to remember – a tragic loss to artists – but apparently one can be trained to grab hold of them. In their lab, the Greens interrupt the students at various times during their feedback training, especially during periods of theta, to ask what was going through their minds. Four of the eight members of their pilot group gradually learned to increase the proportion of their theta waves and also to report on their mental images, after which they would go back into theta. The Greens hope that the students, and other people, will learn to do so as well.

Like stereo buffs, the devotees of bio-feedback develop certain routines or rites. I watched the Greens wire up their daughter, Pat, who has followed the family pattern by becoming a psychologist. Pat had come in for a regular session with the theta-wave pilot group. First Mrs Green parted her daughter's long hair at the back, carefully marked a spot on her scalp (one inch above the inion, a small rise on the back of the head, then half an inch to the right, on the occipital, or visual, area), and applied some whitish electrode paste. Then she rubbed the spot vigorously with a wooden manicure stick until the skin around the paste became bright pink. The paste, she explained, is just an abrasive that is used to help the electrode 'make a good contact'. This was followed by a dab of sticky clay, to prevent the electrode from slipping. The electrode itself, a small flat metal disc with a dangling wire, was then placed securely in the clay. Other devices with trailing wires were attached to three of Pat's fingers, an ear lobe, her wrist, her chest, her left cheekbone, and a spot over her right eyebrow, to give the lab complete records on her temperature, blood-flow, respiration and eye movements. All the wires then had to be tested. Naturally some adjustments were necessary. It took a good forty-five minutes of tinkering, but finally Pat was ready. Reclining on a comfortable chair in a softly lighted, quiet room, she started out with some exercises in concentration. Shortly afterwards, she lay down on a couch next to her chair and began to produce long trains of alpha – regular wavy lines with a characteristic pattern of small, large, then decreasing amplitude, repeated many times. For extended periods she produced nearly 100 per cent alpha; nothing else happened for the next hour. The nervous pens of the recording machines scribbled on pages and pages of folded graph paper, which piled up on the floor, resembling a large accordion. I found it rather boring to watch such voluminous records being turned out. Though Pat's production of alpha waves was high, their frequency did not change and she had almost no theta. It was a disappointment for me – people who try this kind of training should be prepared for it – but Pat seemed quite elated by her experience, despite her lack of theta.

If the Greens had any doubts that some people can, in fact, produce theta waves at will, these were dispelled by the Swami's visit. The Swami – H. H. Swami Rama, forty-five years old, a student of yoga in northern India since the age of four – had been sent to the United States by his guru to tell the West about the effects of yogic training. He spoke good English, but knew hardly anyone in this country and had arrived in Topeka by letting things take care of themselves: a business executive whom he had met in San Francisco had invited him to lecture in Minneapolis, where a man in the audience, a psychiatrist who had trained at Menninger, happened to remember reading about Dr Green's experiments. It took just one long-distance call to make a happy match, and soon the Swami was on his way to the Greens' lab.

The first thing the Swami did was make one half of his right palm 10 degrees warmer than the other half. 'Be attentive, I will do something,' he had announced just before he began. As the Greens watched, one part of his palm slowly flushed as if it had just been slapped, even though the Swami remained completely motionless. Simultaneously, the meter that indicated temperature on that side shot up. It is hard enough to make one hand warmer than the other, Dr Green told me, but to control with such precision the two arteries leading to one palm seemed almost unbelievable. The Swami said it was more difficult than stopping his heart, which he could also do, as he demonstrated the following day. First he made his heart slow down from seventy-five to fifty beats per minute. Then, suddenly, he produced an atrial flutter, during which his heart beat so rapidly that it could no longer pump blood. This is the kind of flutter that normally results in fainting or death. He maintained this state for seventeen seconds, apparently unharmed, and immediately afterwards went off to a lecture. 'My heart is my toy,' the Swami said, with some pleasure. He had played with it all his life, and if he wished he could enter a state much like hibernation, in which all his vital processes would be slowed down.

The Swami carefully examined the lab's equipment, which seemed to impress him. When it was time to record his brain waves, he allowed the electrodes to be placed on his scalp and sat down in the experimental room – but he produced only the fast, active beta waves. Day after day, for two weeks, he appeared unable to relax or meditate. The Greens were completely baffled by this, and the Swami looked miserable. Finally he blurted, 'These two weeks have been wasted, just wasted!' When Dr Green asked him why, the Swami said he'd been worrying too much. 'If only you hadn't told me that the polygraph paper cost $16 a box!' He couldn't bear to think of that large quantity of expensive paper coming out of the machines and piling up on the floor, wasted on him. The Greens assured him that this would not bankrupt the project. Relieved, the Swami lay down again, and fifteen minutes later said he was ready. After some trains of alpha waves, he produced a high volume of theta – 75 per cent of his brain activity for five minutes, an exceptionally high percentage. The following day he produced even slower waves, the delta waves of deep sleep, while remaining fully conscious. 'I couldn't believe it, but he did – and he was not asleep, even though he snored,' says Dr Green. 'He reported 90 per cent of the test sentences Alyce read him, which is better than I could do, and I thought I was wide-awake!'

Asked how he did it, the Swami credited concentration. 'Alpha waves are nothing,' he said, meaning that they were very easy – he simply thought of nothing during that time. Theta waves came when he stilled his conscious mind and brought the unconscious forward. Delta waves, which he called 'yogic sleep', resulted from stilling many parts of his brain at the same time. They were particularly refreshing – in fifteen minutes he could get an hour's worth of good sleep.

As soon as the Swami learned which of his internal states corresponded to the names alpha, theta and delta he could predict with complete accuracy which brain waves he would produce.

This at least showed the extent to which brain-wave control is possible after long yogic training. How much can be achieved by the average person after a relatively short period of bio-feedback training, however, remains an open question. 'Training the body is like training a dog,' says Dr Green. 'You need to fix its attention firmly and hold it long enough.' The curare used in Dr Miller's lab may have been so effective because it cut off all feedback from the skeletal muscles of animals, thereby eliminating distractions. Are there less drastic ways of speeding up feedback training for human beings? Researchers at Rockefeller University are now looking into several possibilities. One way might be to have the computer monitor many different parts of the subject's body simultaneously, to make sure that he is never rewarded for an indirect response. Dr Miller also suggests trying hypnosis, to produce relaxation and to increase the emotional content of the signal that acts as a reward.

There is some question, too, whether bio-feedback training can change people quickly and profoundly enough to be of real therapeutic value outside of the laboratory. Can a person who is seriously ill with heart disease or hypertension actually rely on his new powers of self-control? Or will they desert him in time of crisis? After all, even the Swami found it hard to concentrate while he was anxious about causing what seemed to him a monstrous waste. Bio-feedback's major contribution to medicine may be in the early prevention of disease, in re-educating people before they cause permanent damage to their internal organs.

It might also lead to a healthier way of life. At the University of Colorado Medical Center, Thomas Budzynski, a psychologist, has started re-educating insomniacs by training them to produce slow brain waves. Before giving them E E G feedback, he trains them to relax their forehead muscles through feedback from a different instrument, the electromyograph (E M G). Learning to relax these muscles produces a general relaxation, which he considers a prerequisite for slow-alpha and theta rhythms. Two of his three pilot patients learned to fall asleep readily in this way. Dr Budzynski hopes that millions of people will give up barbiturates and tranquillizers, replacing them with feedback training. He expects theta feedback to speed up psychotherapy by giving patients freer access to previously repressed thoughts, and he points out that anyone who wants a good look at his inner world might benefit from such training.

There can be no quarrel with these attempts at self-education and self-control. However, some well-financed researchers, many of them working for the Department of Defense, have been developing a very different approach to bio-feedback. Their goal is simply to improve the performance of men in combat and other emergencies. They speak the language of strict behaviourism: they refer to 'modification of behaviour through operant conditioning', 'optional schedules of reinforcement' and other terms taken from standard methods of training rats. Although personnel are to be trained in self-control, it is always in the interest of a mission rather than for their own sake – somewhat like teaching soldiers to obey whenever they hear an order.

The Advanced Research Programs Agency of the Defense Department (A R P A) sponsors what is probably the most ambitious programme of bio-feedback research in America, interesting work which may prove of great value if it is not misused.

It includes, for instance, a project started by Dr Jan Berkhout of UCLA's Brain Research Institute, a clever and extremely verbal young psychiatrist who had done some previous work on electrical stimulation of the brains of mental patients. At the Institute he traced the telltale EEGs of normal people when they found certain questions stressful (e.g., 'Do you masturbate?'), to develop a more accurate measure of stress than the lie-detector. Now he is trying 'to condition or enhance' brain-wave patterns that are associated with good performance.

Dr Berkhout told me that he 'violently disagrees' with those who see feedback as the gateway to states of transcendental meditation. 'My own bias is an interest in end performance, not in states of being or conversation with cosmic spirits,' he declared. His present project involves comparing EEG patterns from two different areas of the head, to see how they are related during perception or learning. Some work with monkeys indicates that the best time to assimilate and store new visual information may be when brain waves from the visual area of the cortex are synchronized with those from the visual part of the reticular system, the system that produces arousal. Such synchrony is called 'coherence', and if it turns out that human beings, too, learn best during such coherence, he will try to train people to produce more of it. This training should allow soldiers, and others, to increase their learning ability at will.

Other ARPA goals are to train soldiers to heighten their senses of sight, hearing and smell through bio-feedback, so as to 'avoid ambush and seek out enemy forces and equipment in the field'; to monitor their own alertness, so they can avoid becoming drowsy or inattentive while on guard duty; to control fear; to control pain by regulating the action of fibres in the spinal cord; and to control body temperature – not for relaxation, but for quite specific reasons, such as reducing the swelling and pain of injuries (by cooling) or improving underwater performance by raising the temperature of hands and feet in spite of the cold. ARPA is also concerned about the chronic sleep-loss suffered by so many infantrymen. One group of researchers under contract to the agency is studying whether E E G feedback could teach men to fall asleep more rapidly, so as to make the most of the time they have, while another group aims to find out whether sleep is necessary at all in such conditions – perhaps some state between sleep and rest, which still permitted some kind of vigilance, might be more beneficial.

Even if all these goals were attainable, which is doubtful, there remains the problem of how large numbers of soldiers would be taught to reach them. A R P A has worried about this. Learning self-control takes work and concentration – would the average recruit go to all this trouble just to see a signal that he is doing well? Would a beep be an adequate reinforcement? To be on the safe side, A R P A is looking into the possibility of giving men more concrete rewards for good performance on the feedback machines.

And so this tool of self-mastery, bio-feedback, could become just another, more efficient instrument of mass conditioning.

The difference between operant conditioning and self-education through bio-feedback is sometimes elusive, but it is important: it's merely a question of who is at the controls. In operant conditioning, the experimenter decides on tasks, rewards and punishments, and the subject may not even know that he is being changed. In self-education, a person learns to bring a normally unconscious process under conscious control and gains an extra measure of freedom.

In B. F. Skinner's opinion, we have no choice but to use operant conditioning, in one form or another, to change people's behaviour. He believes this is the only way to ensure peace without repression. Disagreeing, most of the researchers involved in bio-feedback believe that man can change himself through voluntary action. He can reshape his personality, improve his health, in a sense remake his world through bio-feedback.

The possibilities seem nearly unlimited. In Detroit an E E G researcher, Dr Ernst Rodin, has been studying a whole realm of high-frequency brain waves not normally recorded by the standard E E G machines. Since they appear related to the activity of the deeper brain centres, they may lead to important advances in bio-feedback training. In Los Angeles Dr Barry Sterman has isolated several interesting brain rhythms that previously had no name. When he trained cats to increase their production of these rhythms (by offering them milk as a reward), their behaviour changed radically. One group of cats, which he rewarded for what he called the 'sensorimotor rhythm' (12 to 16 cycles per second, from the sensory and motor areas of the cortex), became motionless, as if frozen into stage attitudes. This training had specific advantages: it led to unusually peaceful, unbroken sleep, slowed down the cats' heart rates, and gave them exceptional resistance to certain drugs. Instead of going into convulsions after being exposed to a poisonous compound used in rocket fuels, for instance, these cats took on odd, rigid postures that seemed to ward off the seizures – even three months after their training. This is a clear indication that epileptics may someday learn to control their seizures through bio-feedback.

Another Sterman experiment suggests the fascinating possibility that people may learn to tap their own brains' pleasure centres to produce contentment on demand, without surgery. Dr Sterman had noticed that a certain rhythm appeared in the brain waves of cats right after they received a milk reward and while they were drinking the milk, but never when the cats were too hungry to feel good. It seemed related to their feelings of satiety or enjoyment. He then set out to condition some cats to produce more of this rhythm (a slow wave, 4 to 12 cycles per second, which encompasses theta and most of alpha and which he dubbed the 'post-reinforcement rhythm'). He soon discovered that the more of this rhythm they produced, the less they cared about their milk rewards. They just lay down in the conditioning chamber, their eyes closed, purring, as if in a state of bliss.

For people who experience little pleasure in life such training might be a revelation. It could lead to profound changes in personality, turning a normally tense or grouchy person into one who is fulfilled and well disposed. Possibly this sort of training in early childhood might also reduce the 'fight-or-flight' reactions that so often cause aggressive behaviour and violence in later life.

Bio-feedback is a very new field of research, and it is moving along with explosive speed in many directions. 'We are now embarked on a historic search into our interior to see what has always before been hidden to man,' Gardner Murphy told members of the American Psychiatric Association recently. 'It is a shocking possibility. What shall we see? Are we prepared, really, to face the tremendous blinding flash that's going to come?'

Along with all the discoveries of what our brain, our muscles, and our autonomic nervous system are doing, Dr Murphy warned, will come some larger questions – some very sticky, complicated philosophical issues, like the nature of individuality – which now lie half-concealed in the research reports. Though the notion that we can't observe the process of thinking is quite old, it may no longer be true. 'What with feedback, and slow motion of all sorts, and tremendous gains in equipment, so that what is little becomes enormously big to the observer, perhaps before very long the little indirect awarenesses – such as when I become aware that my words aren't clear, I must hurry, I mustn't overstate my case, and so forth – all these little phases of thought will be right there on the panel.' It may even be possible to observe evidence of the will, or at least of decision-making, and the final confirmation of an act of will.

'There is only the limit of our own ingenuity,' he declared. While some of the claims now being made by the bio-feedback researchers may turn out to have been overbold, Dr Murphy concluded, most of them will prove not to have been bold enough.

5 Drugs: the easiest way to change the brain

You are told that you will have a 'peak' experience of ecstasy and overwhelming beauty, an experience that may change your life. You walk into a comfortable living-room. You greet the psychotherapist, whom you have come to know quite well in the past two weeks; he is now your friend and will soon be your guide.

You lie down on a sofa, next to a stereo set and some inspirational records: harp music, the *Saint Cecilia* Mass, *Death and Transfiguration*. You receive an injection of L S D. Then you put on eye shades to blot out all images but those conjured up within you. You clamp on earphones to intensify the effects of the music. And you try to let go.

This is no illegal trip with black-market drugs, but a carefully monitored session of 'psychedelic peak therapy', during which, the doctor hopes, you will have a profound mystical experience. If you do find religion in this way, you may be cured of what ails you – alcoholism, heroin addiction, neurosis. Even if you don't go all the way, if you don't feel 'reborn' or united with God, you may still gain many of the benefits of psychotherapy, despite the relatively short period of treatment, because of the way the sessions are structured.

Almost anything can happen under L S D, the most powerful psychedelic drug known to man. Psychedelic means 'mind-opening', and L S D opens the mind so that everything is accepted uncritically: spectres from one's unconscious, as well as noises or phrases from one's immediate surroundings. Even a speck of LSD makes one extremely suggestible. It breaks down the boundaries between one's self and others, inducing hallucinations. Their content, however, depends more on the setting than on the drug. This is why the therapist plays a decisive role during LSD sessions at the Maryland State Psychiatric Research Center in Spring Grove Hospital, Baltimore, one of the few centres still allowed to do research with this controversial drug. Well before the session, the therapist prepares the patient to expect an overwhelming transcendental experience. He gains his trust. He encourages the patient to let himself be completely swept into the experience when it comes. He promises to stay with him for the full ten or twelve hours of the drug's effect.

On the big day, fresh flowers are brought into the treatment room. A hand mirror, pictures of the patient's family, and carefully selected musical records are provided as possible props. The therapist is then ready to stage-manage the event. For a long and gruelling day he will sit next to the patient, guide him, reassure him when necessary, have him sit up and talk at times without either music or eye shades, ask him leading questions, help him interpret what he sees, hold his hand, sometimes even hug him if he goes through a moment of terror.

The peak experience, if it occurs at all, usually comes around the third or fourth hour after the intake of LSD. The therapist then attempts to stabilize it, so that the patient remains in an elevated mood for the rest of the session. Success means that the danger of panic or other upsetting reactions is over. On the following day, patient and therapist get together again to review what happened. Intensive therapy, without further LSD, continues for a few more weeks.

In their work with hard-core confirmed alcoholics, psychiatrists at the Maryland centre have found that roughly a third of the patients who were given large doses of LSD achieved profound psychedelic peak reactions, generally of a religious nature. These experiences apparently shook them out of their character-

istic alienation and negativism. Here is how one man described
it:

'Images began to flash through my mind,' he wrote. 'They
were so fast, however, that I couldn't catalogue anything . . . I
lost all sense of time . . . I suddenly saw myself near the bottom
of a huge, filthy pit. It seemed to be bottomless and was crawl-
ing with horrible things such as octopi and enormous, odd-
shaped frogs. I tried to crawl my way out of the pit and finally
got near the top. Looking down, it was horrible . . . Huge vats
and casks containing whisky were being poured into this slimy
pit. It seemed that all the whisky in the world was being
dumped there. I began to cry. A feeling of deep guilt and remorse had come over me. The doctor had me sit up. In discussion with him, I realized the significance of this episode for my
own experience with alcohol. After my crying spell, I felt relieved and cleaner inside.

'Once again I reclined on the couch. The music became
more meaningful to me . . . A tremendous feeling of exaltation
came over me. It kept growing in intensity. I felt rapture and
ecstasy. Each moment I thought I had reached the zenith of
rapture and joy; then the intensity and ecstasy would increase . . .'

Later on, the therapist handed him a mirror. 'I looked,'
wrote the patient, 'but I didn't like what I saw. As I watched,
to my utter horror, my image in the mirror began to age. My
face became older and worn. I saw my skull disintegrate and
turn into ashes, and the ashes were me. In shock and horror, I
turned away from the mirror. The doctor reminded me that
what I had seen had come from me, that it reflected some aspect
of myself. Perhaps I feared that what was in me could lead only
to waste and ruin. He urged me to confront the fear, since I
had already discovered much in myself of value. I understood.
He encouraged me to look again in the mirror. This time I saw
my face in its normal state, and as I did, I realized how deeply
afraid I had always been. I knew that I had long been running
from this fear, but that I would run no longer . . .

'Sometime after this, when I was reclining again, I felt the presence of God and a warm sense of compassion enveloped me. The sense of God that came over me was unlike anything I had ever known. I thought again of how deeply I loved my wife . . . I felt that I could never be the same man again. I felt pure, holy and clean . . . This was the most satisfying and majestic day in my life.'

Eighteen months after their L S D sessions, half of the alcoholics in an experimental high-dose group were still abstaining from liquor – an extraordinarily high proportion, compared with the 10 to 20 per cent recovery rates achieved through other forms of treatment. However, it is not yet clear how much the L S D actually contributed, since a control group of alcoholics who received only small doses of the drug, more like a placebo (50 micrograms, as opposed to 450 micrograms), responded nearly as well. Perhaps the key factor was their belief in their own change.

'We knew that alcoholics who have religious conversions give up drinking,' said Dr Stanislav Grof, the director of psychiatric research at the centre. 'We knew that high doses of L S D are very conducive to conversion. So we expected dramatic changes in the people who had received high doses. But some of them didn't have profound experiences, while others with low doses did.' I asked Dr Grof why he hadn't given any of the patients true placebos, without any L S D in them, for a better experiment. 'We promised them a very unusual experience,' he replied softly. 'We didn't want to disappoint them.' Furthermore, the cat would have been out of the bag at once, he explained: without any sensory changes at all, the patients would be totally let down, and the therapists would know the truth immediately.

Dr Grof has personally conducted over 2,000 psychedelic sessions. Since he began working with L S D in his native Czechoslovakia sixteen years ago, he has treated schizophrenics, sexual deviates, addicts, neurotics, people with severe depressions, people with psychosomatic disorders and 'normal' volunteers ranging from priests to painters and psychiatrists in training. He has taken L S D himself, so as to learn its effects at first hand, and, though he was not at all mystically inclined before, developed religious insights as a result. He clearly believes in the power of the drug. This may help to explain his high rate of success in inducing psychedelic peak experiences, while his success in turn maintains his enthusiasm at a high level. For this reason, and because of the enormous controversy still surrounding L S D, an independent team of researchers, who had never taken psychedelics and who had no information on who had received which dose, was called in to rate the alcoholics after treatment. Their assessment proved fairly close to that of the therapists themselves. They confirmed, for instance, that the patients with the highest percentage of abstinence from alcohol were also those who had had the most profound psychedelic experiences.

When L S D is used merely as a medicine, without all the anticipation, guidance and support provided by psychedelic peak therapy, it does not seem to help alcoholics at all. The Maryland research group, which includes Dr Albert Kurland, Director of the centre, Dr Charles Savage and Dr Sanford Unger, sees L S D as a potent 'enhancer' of psychotherapy, rather than as therapy itself. It believes that L S D is quite safe when taken in this framework, despite the 'bad trips' (severe psychotic reactions) associated with abuse of the drug. Should any patient react so badly during a session that the psychiatrist's reassurance does not help, the doctor can generally stop it with tranquillizers. Only one such case occurred in work with over 200 alcoholics.

The same approach is now being tried with other groups that conventional therapy cannot reach: heroin addicts and people who are dying of cancer. One year after their psychedelic treatment, 24 per cent of the heroin addicts still maintained total abstinence from the drug, a very respectable figure for this particularly stubborn disorder.

Patients approaching death from cancer are perhaps the

loneliest people on earth – their deep depression, pain and hopelessness are sometimes so hard to bear that even their nearest relatives withdraw psychologically, creating a vicious cycle in which the patient becomes ever lonelier and more depressed. Medicine's heroic efforts to keep such persons alive longer have not been matched by efforts to improve the quality of their final months and days. About a decade ago, a Chicago physician, Dr Eric Kast, tried using LSD to help them. He reported that it not only relieved their pain, but in some cases also lifted their depression. He did not, however, combine it with psychotherapy. The Maryland centre did. A moving videotape of an LSD session with a terminal patient, a middle-aged labourer identified only as Jessie, shows the results.

Jessie had a terminal case of skin cancer. At the start of the session he can be seen with a desperate look on his face, complaining about the pain that gives him no respite, despite his many pills. 'It don't stop!' he says. 'I want to be occupied, but I can't do anything. I can't eat. I cry. It hurts me so bad I *got* to cry, I can't help it.' Dr Grof and a psychiatric nurse try to make him comfortable on the sofa. Dr Grof advises him not to keep any feelings bottled up during the therapy, but to let them all out. Then Jessie receives an injection of LSD and lies down, wearing the eye shades. After a while he sits up, choking (because of his illness). He spits into a bowl. The nurse helps him lie down again, but he is clearly frantic. 'Try to really listen to the music,' counsels Dr Grof. 'Let it carry you – beyond the pain, beyond the choking!' Jessie tries. In a gravelly voice he begins to tell about his vision: a junkyard full of tin cans. He is clearly unaware of its symbolism. He talks about Jehovah, and about a huge ball of fire through which he has to go. He cries. Then he describes someone being set free. 'When your body goes, you're destroyed all over,' he says slowly, towards the end of the session. 'You're back to what you started from . . . but your soul'll be living. You don't know what you'll be in the next earth, when you live again . . . You can be something else, you know, whether an animal or other . . . You just got to take what comes in life. You just got to put up with it.' He seems calmer, more reconciled to his fate.

The night after his L S D session, Jessie slept better, and the following day he announced that 'now I'm living through God'. In answer to a question from Dr Grof, he said, 'Of course I never thought of this stuff before, till I went through all this.'

Another videotape shows a thirty-nine-year-old woman who has an inoperable cancer of the stomach. Under the influence of L S D, she seems to go through every possible emotion, alternately panting, sobbing, writhing, licking her lips, moaning and smiling as the music surges on. She was 'in another century' she tells the therapist, hugging him for comfort. She saw India, Egypt and Mexico, none of which she had ever visited. 'The colours and textures were indescribable,' she says. 'But it doesn't matter if you can describe it or not – it's just there!' 'Has it been a day or half an hour?' she asks after ten hours have elapsed. She seems amazed at everything that happened to her while her eyes were closed. Later on she has a blissful look on her face – the so-called psychedelic afterglow – and greets her husband with a radiant smile when he walks in.

In a way she was lucky: the L S D therapy came quite early in her illness, lifting her spirits so effectively that she remained strong and able to walk far longer than her doctor had expected. She also lived several months beyond the predicted time.

Dr Grof feels no qualms about inducing religious experiences, through drugs, in people who might otherwise never have any. 'I don't think we are *inducing* religion,' he said. 'I believe it's an intrinsic part of human nature. The only question is whether or not we get in touch with it.' Psychedelic drugs don't have specific effects like those of penicillin or digitalis, he continues. All they can do is activate deep unconscious processes. 'And if you have a dying patient, *anything* that eases their suffering is good. That's one case in which you can have no philosophical objections!' Roughly a third of these patients improve dramatically after the psychedelic treatment, while another third show some improvement and the rest remain unchanged.

A colleague of Dr Grof's offers another view of the religious experiences: in our culture, when a person under L S D suddenly feels suffused with love or ecstatic awe, religion may offer the only framework for labelling or interpreting it. Given the right dose of psychedelic drugs, the appropriate expectations and a conducive setting, almost anyone may have a deeply mystical experience – the kind of illumination which Christians call a beatific vision and Zen Buddhists call satori. It may no longer be necessary to be a saint like Teresa of Avila, or to undergo extremes of self-mortification.

As in hypnosis, the actual changes come from within. The therapist or hypnotist merely draws them out, acting as a sort of guide to the process of auto-suggestion. Even without a hypnotist, placebos such as sugar pills can greatly relieve the pain of approximately 35 per cent of patients who are recovering from surgery, as was proved repeatedly in tests conducted by Dr Henry Beecher, Harvard's famous professor of research in anaesthesia. One's own expectations may well be the most powerful factor in any reaction to non-lethal doses of mind-changing drugs.

These expectations vary according to one's culture. Dr Solomon Snyder, a professor of psychiatry and pharmacology at Johns Hopkins University, likes to tell of the lovely Indian lab technician who once worked for him. As a little girl, she had been very thin, and her parents worried about it. They took her to one of Bombay's finest physicians, asking for medicine to make her plumper. The doctor prescribed marijuana – a glass of it in liquid form, called *bhang*, before every meal – to increase her appetite. She drank it faithfully three times a day for years until, at seventeen, she was judged sufficiently seductive and allowed to stop. But since it was merely a medicine, and no one had told her it could change her mood in any way, she never felt the least bit intoxicated or otherwise affected by it.

The Maryland group is unusual in seeing L S D as the means to a mystical experience. Other researchers use it either to simulate psychosis (in order to study the mental illness), or as an aid to deep self-analysis, without any mystical overlay. The transcendental or blissful state sometimes produced by L S D merely stands in the way of the primary goal, self-analysis, declares Dr John Lilly, who began taking L S D in the mid-1960s. If one stops at religious beliefs, no analytical progress in further analysis can be made, he writes in his recent book *Programming and Meta-programming in the Human Biocomputer*, which was published by the Whole Earth Catalog. 'These beliefs are "analysis dissolvers" . . . One of these very powerful evasions is a hedonistic acceptance of things as they are, with conversion of most of them to a pleasant glow. Another similar evasion is deferring discussion of such basic issues until one's "life after death" . . . After having been through some of the most innermost depths of self, a result is that they are only one's own beliefs . . . There is nothing else but stored experience.'

This 'stored experience' is what Dr Lilly wants to reach. A man of wide-ranging interests – he is a neurophysiologist and biophysicist as well as a psychoanalyst – he had previously studied the brains of dolphins (see Chapter 1). Before using L S D he experimented with another technique which also facilitates brain-washing: sensory deprivation. In the 1950s Donald Hebb of McGill University had discovered that when a person stops receiving signals from his senses his brain starts playing tricks on him. Volunteers who lay in bed for more than one day with their eyes covered by a translucent visor, their hands wrapped in gloves and their ears plugged up, began to hallucinate. Those who stood it for as long as four days became so deranged that for a while they could not do the simplest tests. It seemed that without a constant flow of information about the world, the brain could not function properly – which is why solitary confinement is a major tool of brain-washing. Dr Lilly decided that the hallucinations came from the brain's attempt to maintain its activity at a normal pace. In the absence of sound or other stimuli from the external world, the sensory cortex used material from programme storage and from internal body sources of excitation. The person undergoing sensory deprivation then interpreted his brain's activity as if the excitation came from outside, from the real world, when in fact it came from inner sources. As Dr Lilly saw it, however, the experience did not present a threat. Instead, it offered a new opportunity to study the subconscious, the 'metaprogrammes' underlying the programmes by which one normally operates. He soon tried it out on himself.

A decade later, he added L S D to the experience of sensory deprivation in an attempt to reach even further into his subconscious. Immersing himself, naked, into a tank of water at body temperature so as to block out all physical sensations, he floated as if in a void, in silence and total darkness. Then he took L S D. After a period of fear, he found it immensely pleasurable. 'One of the pitfalls of L S D-25 experience,' he declared, 'is exactly this: one has the power now to stay in an expanded state of pleasure, as it were, for several hours. This can become quite seductive and one can become quite lazy and return to this state at every opportunity.'

The purpose of all this self-analysis, according to Dr Lilly, is to grow both intellectually and emotionally. 'If successful, one may see one's self operating in improved fashion with other people, as judged by one's self and, much later, as judged by others.' Nevertheless, by most standards his book describing this attempt is so disorganized and jumbled that it falls far below the level of his previous work, and some of his fellow scientists, when asked about him, just shake their heads in bewilderment.

'Candidly considered, one may ask, "May not this substance under these conditions change my brain and mind structure irreversibly out of my control?"' writes Dr Lilly. 'The proper controls on whether or not there are permanent changes in brains have not been done on animals' nor on humans' brains. So there definitely is a risk in this area.'

L S D's primary risk is that, through its distortion of reality, it can trigger off a psychotic reaction. If L S D is taken without supervision, an even more immediate danger is accidental death as the user jumps out of a window, convinced he can fly, or drills a hole in his head 'to release cerebral pressure', as one young man tried to do. However, it is not addictive, except in the way Dr Lilly described.

Although we now know a great deal about how people feel under LSD, its effect on the brain remains unclear. The drug is known to concentrate in the more primitive centres such as the hippocampus (involved in memory), the pineal gland (once a third eye on top of the skulls of early reptiles), and the system concerned with arousal, including the raphe neurons, which are involved in dreaming. LSD also blocks the firing of neurons that respond to 5-hydroxy-tryptamine (5HT), one of the brain's neuro-transmitters. Since the real function of 5HT is unknown, however, this provides only one small piece of the jigsaw puzzle. In the long run LSD may produce some damage, but the evidence is only suggestive. At UCLA, Dr William McGlothin found that some long-term users scored quite low on tests of abstract abilities (such as tests of categories) but did well on tests of verbal abilities. This combination – low abstract and high verbal – often indicates brain damage. In six out of sixteen heavy users of LSD, including the three who took it most frequently, Dr McGlothin found ratios of abstract to verbal scores that made him 'moderately suspicious' of such damage.

Brain chemistry has made tremendous advances in recent decades; or, depending on how you look at it, nothing is yet known about the chemistry of the brain. The best way to measure the field's progress is against the abysmal ignorance of the past. 'Twenty years ago we couldn't say anything about brain chemistry affecting behaviour, except that low brain sugar or low oxygen produced coma,' recalls Dr Daniel Freedman, Chairman of the University of Chicago's psychiatry department. 'Between coma and consciousness, there was nothing. Now the research is beginning to take off.'

The first jolt came with the discovery, in 1943, that the minutest dose of LSD – as little as one three-millionth of an ounce – could produce symptoms similar to insanity. This led to

99

the idea that the psychoses are also produced by tiny amounts of a brain chemical gone awry. Suddenly there was reason to hope for a chemical cure for schizophrenia, depression and other ills.

In 1952 chlorpromazine, the first modern tranquillizing drug, entered the American market. Together with other major tranquillizers such as reserpine, it proved so effective in controlling the symptoms of schizophrenia that mental hospitals began to release their patients in droves. The use of straitjackets and other physical restraints dropped. Lobotomies decreased, and shock treatments became less widespread.

Then came the anti-depressants, a whole class of drugs which rescued thousands of persons from fear, immobility and despair. The anti-depressants were followed by a flood of new psychoactive drugs – anti-anxiety drugs, sedatives and stimulants of various kinds. In addition, lithium was found to control the manic phase of manic-depressive illness. Another chemical, L-Dopa, proved able to reduce the tremors of Parkinsonism.

By any standards, these were extraordinary achievements, allowing millions of people to lead nearly normal lives instead of being confined in institutions. The brain scientists would have good reason to feel very proud of themselves – if it weren't for the fact that they really don't understand how the drugs do what they do.

They have developed a lot of promising clues, however. Most of these involve the brain's neuro-transmitters, the chemicals that carry messages from one neuron to the next, telling it to fire or resist firing. A drug's effect on the brain appears to depend primarily on how it alters the messages carried by specific neuro-transmitters in specific parts of the brain. The chemical code is extremely specific: one kind of neuro-transmitter, acetylcholine, will make a satiated rat start to drink again, for instance, while another transmitter, noradrenaline, applied to exactly the same spot in the rat's hypothalamus, will activate different neurons and compel it to eat.

Before a drug can affect the transmitters in any way, it must cross the blood-brain barrier. This is not an iron curtain, but a series of filters that protect brain tissue from harmful substances in the bloodstream. All chemicals that enter the bloodstream naturally circulate through the brain, in the network of blood vessels that bring it oxygen and nutrients. But very few substances ever pass from these vessels into the surrounding brain tissue. The blood-brain barrier will let them through only if they are highly soluble in such liquid solvents as alcohol or acetone, and if they do not carry a large positive charge.

One chemical that crosses the blood-brain barrier with enormous ease is amphetamine – 'speed'. After seeping from the blood vessels into the surrounding brain tissue, amphetamine multiplies the effects of one of the brain's most interesting neuro-transmitters, noradrenaline (also called norepinephrine), which it closely resembles. Noradrenaline is the transmitter for the sympathetic nervous system, which produces the aroused 'fight-or-flight' response. Not surprisingly, amphetamine makes people alert, excited, hyperactive. It was known as a stimulant long before noradrenaline was found in the brain.

Introduced in the 1930s with the blessings of physicians, amphetamine has been used in inhalers for asthma patients, in the treatment of narcolepsy (an abnormal desire to sleep), in 'pep' pills, in diet pills, by soldiers and truck-drivers who have to stay awake, by students cramming for exams, and only since the late 1960s for the euphoria – the orgasmic 'rush' – it may produce when injected into the veins. It has probably been the most widely and carelessly prescribed addictive drug and, although tighter government regulations have curbed its use in recent years, it remains frequently abused today.

The Japanese were the first to suffer from its effects on a widespread scale. After the Second World War, when Japanese drug companies had large stocks of amphetamine to dispose of (these had originally been intended for workers in munitions factories, to help them produce more), they began advertising amphetamines 'for elimination of drowsiness and repletion of the spirit'. This caught on among the young, and by the mid-

1950s more than 500,000 Japanese had become amphetamine addicts, with at least 50,000 cases of amphetamine psychosis – some of whom are still in the back wards of Japanese mental hospitals. The government became so alarmed that it imposed six-month jail sentences on all who were found in possession of the drug. After this, the epidemic waned, and within three years it was over. It has not flared up since.

In Great Britain, heroin addicts took up amphetamine when their supplies of legal heroin dwindled as a result of new regulations in 1968. Meanwhile adolescents had begun to experiment with amphetamine, and by the late 1960s they were injecting it directly into their bloodstream to obtain the 'rush' for which they needed increasingly large doses. This was a particularly dangerous trend, since large doses produce paranoia and often violence, as Dr P. H. Connell of the Maudsley Hospital in London showed when he provided the first description of amphetamine psychosis in 1958. Alarmed at the growing misuse of the drug, the manufacturers agreed to stop selling injectable amphetamine to anyone except hospital pharmacists. Injectable amphetamine thus disappeared almost overnight, but powdered forms of the drug remained available. These, too, could be injected after being dissolved in water. The Misuse of Drugs Act of 1971 is now putting further pressure on doctors to prevent them from prescribing any form of amphetamine in more than very limited quantities.

America's amphetamine epidemic also began in the late 1960s. Ten thousand million amphetamine pills were produced annually – about fifty for each man, woman and child – and at least half of them were diverted to illegal use.

Most physicians agree that there are only two legitimate uses for amphetamines, both quite rare: to treat narcolepsy and, paradoxically, to calm down certain types of hyperactive children. Nevertheless, American diet doctors continue to dispense amphetamine pills to obese people, especially women, in an effort to reduce their appetite. (British doctors have largely switched to fenfluramine, a related drug which is believed to be non-addictive.) Other physicians prescribe Benzedrine, Dexedrine, or similar pills to athletes or students who want an extra spurt of physical or mental energy. And until injectable amphetamines were banned in the U.S. in the spring of 1973, fashionable doctors injected speed into the veins of some of the nation's most famous public figures – politicians, artists, writers, actors and other jet-setters – not to treat them for disease, but to give them feelings of strength and unbounded confidence. According to a report in the *New York Times* for example, Dr Max Jacobson of New York was known for the unusual quantities of amphetamine he used in his practice. He bought enough of the drug to make a hundred fairly strong doses of 25 milligrams every day. All his patients received large numbers of injections in which various ingredients were mixed: vitamins, hormones and enzymes, as well as amphetamines. He will not reveal which of his patients received amphetamines and which, if any, did not. However, he often talks about his most famous patients: President and Mrs John Kennedy, whom he frequently visited in the White House and with whom he sometimes travelled. 'In 1961, for example, he went with the President to Vienna for the secret meeting with Khrushchev and, Dr Jacobson said in an interview, gave the President injections there,' the *Times* reported. Another physician who treated President Kennedy was outraged by this. 'No President with his finger on the red button has any business taking stuff like that,' he commented.

Amphetamine gives people a chemical boost by releasing noradrenaline at the synapses. It also counteracts the normal 're-uptake' of noradrenaline in the brain. After a neuro-transmitter has done its job of telling a neuron to fire, it must be inactivated in order to prevent it from repeating this order endlessly. Some transmitters, such as acetylcholine, are inactivated by enzymes. Others, such as noradrenaline and dopamine, are inactivated by being taken back by the nerve-endings that released them; amphetamine inhibits this process. The resulting increase in noradrenaline and dopamine in the brain can have different effects, depending on which pathways are stimulated.

Besides its rousing, stimulating effects, amphetamine is known to produce a strange sort of repetitiveness. Speed freaks will perform compulsive, stereotyped acts over and over again, without apparent boredom. Dr Solomon Snyder describes a teenager who counted cornflakes all night long. This stereotyped behaviour seems related to the brain's dopamine tracts, rather than to noradrenaline, judging from recent work by Dr Snyder and his colleagues. Amphetamine psychosis also seems related to dopamine. Furthermore, tranquillizers that block dopamine in the brain relieve both schizophrenia and amphetamine psychosis. Dr Snyder concludes that if researchers succeed in finding a chemical that stimulates *only* the dopamine tracts, they will have a perfect model for studying schizophrenia in animals. On the other hand, a drug that stimulates only the noradrenaline tracts may produce pure, undiluted euphoria, since these tracts go right through the brain's pleasure centres. After an injection of amphetamine, rats that have electrodes in their pleasure centres stimulate themselves even more furiously.

Research on how drugs affect the brain has been greatly advanced by a dazzling Swedish technique that uses fluorescence to trace the neuro-transmitters. At Stockholm's Karolinska Institut, slices of brain tissue were treated with chemicals that caused various transmitters to glow brilliantly under ultraviolet light. This led to entirely new maps of the brain, quite different from those based on anatomy, for it showed that the cells containing specific transmitters form special networks in specific parts of the brain. Noradrenaline glows in bright green. 5HT is yellow. Like the strings of coloured lights seen from an aeroplane window at night, these networks indicate some of the brain's main thoroughfares.

How many thoroughfares there are remains unknown. The kind of neuro-transmitter that tells you instantly to pull your hand off a hot plate may be quite different from the one that causes you to decide you're hungry for Chinese food, points out Dr Floyd Bloom, of the National Institute of Mental Health's Laboratory of Neuropharmacology. Dr Bloom believes that different kinds of information-processing systems are activated by different transmitters.

If he is right, the brain scientists still have a long way to go. 'The noradrenaline-containing cells make up less than 1 per cent of all cells in the brain,' declared Dr Bloom. 'What are the transmitters for the other 99 per cent of nerve cells?' Though researchers have developed good tools to work with noradrenaline and also know something about dopamine, 5HT and acetylcholine, they still have almost no information about amino acids such as GABA, glycine and glutamate, transmitters that are far more prominent in the brain. 'The concentration of these amino acids in the brain is probably one thousand times great than that of noradrenaline or acetylcholine,' said Dr Bloom. 'The transmitters we know how to measure are just the top of the iceberg.

'People say the brain is like a computer. But suppose you found a computer and it did things. Even if you knew how it was wired, could you tell how it worked? Not unless you knew how to speak Fortran or whatever machine language it was programmed in – and nobody knows what the machine language of the brain really is.' Nothing in the brain is ever completely on, nor ever completely off. One can never tell whether some behaviour is the result of the excitation of one group of cells, the inhibition of another, the disinhibition of a third or the result of millions of contradictory influences. 'It's so complicated you can't expect at the beginning to come up with anything close to the final answer,' Dr Bloom said. 'All you can do is to keep looking, and to test out new theories as knowledge expands.'

Practical applications of what we learn about brain chemistry may come well before the theoreticians make much progress. For example, chemical stimulation of the brain is now a real possibility. Recently a group of researchers at Princeton University showed that normally peaceful laboratory-bred rats could be turned into killers by injecting certain drugs into specific parts of their hypothalamus. Apparently the transmitter acetylcholine was responsible for releasing this aggression. The

105

psychologists Bartley Hoebel, Douglas Smith and Melvyn King first located certain cells in the rats' hypothalami where electrical stimulation triggered off a killing attack on any nearby mouse. Then they inserted tiny hollow tubes into the rats' brains, ending near these cells, and tried a variety of drugs. When they poured in a few drops of carbachol, which acts much like acetylcholine, the rats pounced on the mice and killed them with a single hard bite on the back of their necks. This was their first murder – and they had never seen any such killing before. Next the scientists took wild rats that were known for their furious attacks on mice and tried to turn off their killer instinct with drugs. Methyl atropine, they knew, blocks the effects of acetylcholine. With atropine in their brains, the wild rats suddenly became pacifists. They walked up to the mice, sniffed them and followed them around for a while, but they did not kill. Dr Smith finds it conceivable that similar 'pharmacological prevention' could control aggressive behaviour in human beings.

Other practical applications may come from current research on how drugs affect sleep. Man spends the equivalent of twenty years of his life asleep – a state about which much has been learned since the mid-1950s, when scientific research on sleep began. The more one learns, however, the more curious it seems. Far from being a uniform period of quiet, sleep turns out to be a most active time for the brain, a succession of radically different states, each with its characteristic EEG pattern. Throughout the night, in cycles, comes the recurrent period of fast brain waves, quickened heart rate, teeth-grinding, erections (in males of every age, including infants and premature babies), irregular breathing and rapid eye movements, called REM. This is the time of vivid dreaming for all human beings, and perhaps even for animals. A person who is awakened during REM sleep will invariably report a dream, or dream-like thoughts. Awakened only a few minutes after the rapid eye movements cease, he will remember nothing: the dream will have evaporated. Regardless of how much one remembers, however, everyone dreams every night. The REM periods occur roughly every ninety minutes, or about five times a night, and take up about 20 per cent of one's total sleep time.

A strange feature of nearly all mood-changing drugs, particularly amphetamine and barbiturates, is that they radically reduce the amount of REM sleep. Yet REM sleep seems to be essential. Volunteers who are deprived of it by being awakened every time their eyeballs begin to move become very anxious and irritable, prone to hallucinations and temporarily unable to think straight. They also develop an almost irresistible urge to dream. Towards the end of REM-deprivation experiments, the researchers must wake them up more and more frequently, for they fall into the REM state almost as soon as they close their eyes. They seem compelled to fill their deficit of REM. When finally given a chance to sleep undisturbed, they will have an orgy of dreaming – and this after only a few days of REM deprivation. Experiments with cats and rats can be pushed even further. On their first free night after one or two months of REM deprivation, these animals will spend 70 per cent of their total sleep time in a REM state so agitated and intense that it actually resembles convulsive seizures.

Brain scientists are now wondering to what extent the harmful effects of various drugs can be attributed to their destruction of REM sleep. Dr Ian Oswald of the University of Edinburgh believes that the brain repairs itself during REM sleep – an interesting theory in view of the fact that babies spend an enormous amount of time in REM sleep and schizophrenics very little. Dr Chris Evans of the National Physical Laboratory at Teddington, suggests that the main purpose of dreams may be to 'clean up' the brain's current programmes, just as computer programmes are periodically cleaned up to rid them of the clutter of accumulated, obsolete instructions. As circumstances change, computer programmes are constantly modified, but unless the resulting 'junk' is filtered out, the programmes become much less effective or actually break down. Something similar seems to happen when human beings are deprived of dreams. Other scientists have found evidence of some links between the REM state and the brain's supply of 5HT. But whatever the theory all researchers agree that after REM deprivation people suffer in varying degrees from a kind of rebound effect, during which their brain tries desperately to compensate for its loss. Only schizophrenics seem unable to compensate for it.

When people take sleeping pills, they unwittingly starve themselves of REM sleep. After a week or two, when they try to do without pills, they begin to feel the rebound effects: they dream for nearly half the night and sometimes have terrifying nightmares. Naturally they reach for another sleeping pill, and the vicious cycle begins. Soon they find that they cannot do without these pills. They also need increasingly large quantities to get any results. Since large doses of barbiturates act longer than people suppose, it becomes increasingly difficult for them to wake up in the morning. At this point they may try Dexedrine or some other amphetamine to get themselves going. The amphetamine further reduces the incidence of REM sleep, completing the cycle: they are now slaves to 'downers' at night and 'uppers' in the morning. This is how, by handing a patient some perfectly legal sleeping pills, doctors sometimes create sleep disorders instead of curing them – and also how many middle-class addicts are made, especially middle-aged women.

Death may result if the befuddled victim forgets she has already taken a sleeping pill and swallows another, as reportedly happened to Marilyn Monroe and some other film stars. The pills are particularly powerful if taken in combination with alcohol, also a depressant. The brain then slows down so completely that it stops telling the heart to beat or the lungs to breathe, and all body functions come to a halt.

The drugs that are most addictive, such as barbiturates, amphetamine, heroin and alcohol, produce the most violent reactions when they are withdrawn. Usually the reactions are the reverse of the drug's original effects. The withdrawal of alcohol, for instance, causes sudden overactivity of the brain, which may result in the well-known delirium tremens, or D.T.s, complete with pink elephants and other imaginary but terrifying monsters or bugs. Withdrawal of the euphoriant and excitant amphetamines produces almost unbearable depression, often with suicidal impulses. After the feeling of peace gained from barbiturates, the addict may have hallucinations and convulsions when he stops taking the pills.

At autopsy, however, no particular brain damage can be seen from any of these drugs, despite the upheavals they produce. As with mental illness, the effect of mind-changing drugs remains invisible in the brain; at any rate, it cannot be detected with present methods.

The only exception is alcohol. Alcohol seems to produce minute blood clots and haemorrhages in the capillaries that feed the cells of both body and brain. Around each plugged capillary in the brain, some nerve cells die for lack of oxygen. And though most of the body's cells are replaceable, the brain's nerve cells are not – once gone, they are lost forever.

With every single cocktail, we may kill thousands of brain cells. Considering that the adult brain contains some ten thousand million nerve cells, this is not so terrible – hundreds of brain cells die every day for a variety of reasons, anyway. Nevertheless, in heavy drinkers the loss eventually takes its toll. Within a few years they may lose millions of irreplaceable cells, and when the brains of alcoholics are examined at autopsy they often appear shrunken or atrophied. Doctors disagree on what causes this damage, however. Some argue that it results from the alcoholics' notoriously poor nutrition. Others blame the by-products of a damaged liver. To date, there is no direct evidence that alcohol produces primary damage to the brain.

The lack of firm evidence about brain damage from drugs has proved very disappointing to those who seek physical excuses for stiffer legislation against pushers of hard drugs. The social evidence, however, is strong enough: drug abuse, as we all know, can lead to crime, paranoia, death. It is a sort of chemical Russian roulette. Even the softer and legal psychoactive drugs present real dangers, despite the fact that they may be prescribed by a doctor.

While illicit drugs spread through word of mouth, the drug industry spends millions of dollars every year on advertising aimed at physicians. Full-page advertisements in medical journals urge doctors to prescribe drugs for every eventuality: for women who are disturbed by jealousy, or depressed by their wrinkles; for small children who fear the dark; for those who are afraid of going to school; for all who feel anxious.

More prescriptions were written for psychoactive drugs in America last year than there were people in the country, according to J. Maurice Rogers, the research director of the San Francisco Community Mental Health Services. Pointing out that pharmaceutical companies depend on the nation's physicians to sell their prescription drugs, he accused the drug advertisements of being 'grossly irresponsible, especially those that push psychoactive drugs – sedatives, sleeping pills, tranquillizers, energizers and mood-elevators'. Not only do these advertisements make broad, unsupportable claims, but they extend drug usage into areas that call for coping, not for escape through drugs. In that sense psychoactive drugs are not innocent, even when not toxic, according to Dr Robert Seidenberg, Professor of Psychiatry at the State University of New York at Syracuse. 'They tend to create a dependence, to undermine confidence in personal mastery, and they are frequently antithetical to psychotherapy.' Medical societies, too, have become 'drug dependent' he said, because they rely so heavily on advertising by drug companies – the very advertisements which strenuously promote an improper use of drugs.

Partly because of such advertisements, there is a growing tendency to give children pills for anything that comes to the attention of the doctor. It is the easiest way out. If parents are troubled by a child's anxiety, or if they feel unable to meet his demands, the doctor may simply label the child 'disturbed' and prescribe tranquillizers for him.

In its recent report on 'Medicines in the 1990s – A Techno-logical Forecast,' the Office of Health Economics in London has predicted a similar emphasis on drugs in Britain. 'It is likely that by 1990 nearly every individual will be taking psychotropic medicines either continuously or at intervals', it stated.

The more the drug industry expands its definition of what constitutes a medical problem, however, the greater the danger of abuse. It is only a short step from the careless use of mind-changing drugs for the treatment of everyday problems to the use of drugs to control *other* people whose behaviour makes one uncomfortable.

A couple of years ago, the *Washington Post* described how one paediatrician in Omaha, Nebraska, encouraged local doctors to prescribe 'behaviour modification' drugs to as many as 5 to 10 per cent of the 62,000 schoolchildren in that city. The children being given the drugs had been identified by their teachers as 'hyperactive' and unmanageable to the point of disrupting the classroom, reported the *Post*. The drugs were prescribed 'to improve classroom deportment and increase learn-ing potential'. The teachers clearly liked their effect, though some of the parents didn't.

As enthusiasm for the programme increased, 'thousands of elementary school children were walking around with poten-tially dangerous drugs in their pockets and lunch-pails', the newspaper reported. An assistant superintendent of schools said the children 'were trading pills on the school grounds. One kid would say, "Here, you try my yellow one and I'll try your pink one." '

What were these pills? Mostly, amphetamine and Ritalin, a similar drug. Both, when given to adults, would be extremely dangerous and addictive. Both normally act as stimulants. When used with hyperactive children, however – children who jump out of their seats as many as thirty times in five minutes, who keep fidgeting, who throw things and talk, who can't concen-trate – these drugs seem to have the opposite effect.

'The amphetamines quiet them down,' says Dr Solomon

111

Snyder of Johns Hopkins University. 'They become very conscientious. They get tearful if you say a harsh word. And the strange thing is that little kids, weighing no more than eighty pounds, will tolerate doses of amphetamines that would be an overdose for an adult. The drug would make *us* hyperactive on ten milligrams. Children, who are usually hypersensitive to drugs, can tolerate forty milligrams per day and seem no worse for it.' Highly respected psychiatrists, such as Dr Leon Eisenberg of Harvard University, claim that no child has become addicted as a result of such treatment. Instead, in case after case, behaviour problems has disappeared and school grades shot up.

The only trouble with this approach is that hyperactivity can have a wide variety of causes, including social deprivation, emotional problems, psychosis and poor teaching, as well as the 'minimal brain dysfunction' for which the drugs were originally prescribed. It is a symptom, not a disease. And even in a first-rate hospital such as Johns Hopkins, where children are screened very carefully before being given the drugs, some children get worse after taking them. 'We had a little girl here who took one pill and became crazy for two days,' Dr Snyder recalled. 'She saw icicles and tigers.' Fortunately, reactions to amphetamine are very rapid, and the treatment is simply to stop taking such pills. The little girl recovered. But doctors cannot predict what any particular child's reaction will be. 'Ultimately it may be possible to tell more accurately who fits into this diagnostic category,' Dr Snyder said. Which category? 'Hyperactive-that-responds-to-these-drugs,' he replied with a smile.

Omaha was not alone: some 200,000 children in the United States were, and probably are, being given drugs to prevent them from fidgeting or disrupting their classroom. Many of them were poor and black. Some black parents began to complain that the schools were trying to drug their children into submission. Various other parents said they resented the pressure being put on them by teachers to go to a doctor and ask for these drugs for their children.

In hearings before a subcommittee of the House Committee

on Government Operations, a congressman asked, 'Who makes a decision in these programmes as to whether a child has hyper-kinesis or is just a bored, bright, creative, pain-in-the-neck kid?' He did not seem satisfied with the reply that a medical team, or at least one doctor, had to be involved, since all too often the children were first picked out by the schools. One of the wit-nesses pointed out that between one-and-a-half and four mil-lion children between the ages of three and twelve were potential recipients of such drugs, and that their use was 'zooming'. Yet the follow-up studies of hyperactive children who have used them involved only sixty-seven children. 'How do you draw the line?' asked Representative John Wydler of New York. 'If you read all the good results of giving these children drugs you wonder, maybe if you gave every child a little bit of it, they might be all better off. They might all become more docile or more co-operative or something of this nature . . . It would help them be more attentive in school. This seems to be almost the logic of where you will go once you start down this road.' The psychiatrist under questioning replied that it was a matter of degree, and that he had enough experience to make a judgement about it. But the uneasiness remains, since most children with hyperactivity show no sure signs of brain damage. Nothing sets them apart from others except their behaviour. To a large ex-tent, then, they can be given drugs for the convenience of their parents or their teachers. This may produce a new form of addic-tion. All we know is that here, in a small pill, is instant relief, instant satisfaction – *for the caretaker*. Unlike other forms of addiction, in this case the pill must be swallowed by somebody else.

This kind of abuse is well known in mental hospitals and nursing homes where nurses give their charges large doses of tranquillizers to keep them quiet and easy to handle. Usually the doctors co-operate by writing out blanket orders for drugs, which can be used at the nurses' discretion, whether the patients need them or not. Far from helping these patients, especially if they are old people who require an incentive to move about, such massive use of drugs tends to turn them into vegetables.

Giving drugs to children who make trouble in school may help some of them to settle down and concentrate, thus preventing further difficulties. But in other cases it may mask problems that could be solved through social measures. Furthermore, the amphetamines' effect is not at all clear.

The hyperactive children who become very neat, quiet and orderly after taking amphetamine may have something in common with the adult speed freaks who keep repeating stereotyped acts without apparent boredom. In both cases, the dopamine-sensitive cells in their brains seem to be involved, rather than the noradrenaline pathways. However, nobody yet understands why these children's reaction is otherwise paradoxical – why they become calm instead of still more excited. Since the hyperactive symptoms tend to disappear in all such children after they reach puberty, hormones may be involved in some still inexplicable fashion.

The drugs may also interfere with the children's appetites and sleep, particularly with their REM periods. All this is bad enough, but there must be other short- and long-range effects we don't yet know about. There can also be a strong placebo effect, both on the child and on his teachers. One witness at the House investigation told of a boy whose teacher had picked him out as hyperactive. His doctor had prescribed Ritalin, and his parents had pretended to accept this, although in fact they never gave the child any drugs at all. Since the teacher believed the boy was taking the pills, she started treating him differently and in a short time his grades improved.

All drugs have multiple and complex effects, especially the mind-changing drugs. The effects that drug companies like best are generally called the main effects. Other changes, however big, are labelled 'side effects'. Should these 'side effects' prove even more interesting and powerful than the main effects, the drug is simply relabelled, as has happened to many of the best-known tranquillizers.

The idea that a 'magic bullet' type of drug can seek out a specific target in the body and destroy it has long held much appeal in medicine. Something of the same notion persists in the ads which promise that Librium will 'reduce anxiety', that Compoz will 'calm the nerves', and that Elavil will 'lift depression'. In fact, according to the psychiatrist Henry Lennard and his colleagues at the University of California School of Medicine at San Francisco, such specificity is a fiction created by the labelling process. Research does not support a purely physiological view of the emotions, and 'drugs alone do not trigger off such specific affective reactions as fear, anger, depression, joy, and the like'. The drugs only produce a state of arousal, or a general 'priming' of the body. How a person interprets these changes depends both on cues from the environment and on his own past experiences. Instead of being a passive recipient of drugs, each person actively builds his own reality.

With some drugs, the social context is the most important variable: for example, LSD and other hallucinogens make people extremely suggestible. Large doses of amphetamine sometimes produce such paranoia and aloofness that their victims are practically unreachable by any human being. But there is always this interaction between drug, social situation and mental set.

The brain scientists must bear some blame for failing to make this clear. People who take LSD should know that their 'trips' will, in a sense, brainwash them, and that whatever influences they are exposed to during that time may become imprinted on them for life. They should know that, of all drugs, the amphetamines are the most rapidly addictive, and they should be made aware of the alternatives.

As Dr René Dubos has observed, human beings have always taken drugs – coffee, tea, wine, maté. 'I have been told that Gandhi took reserpine very frequently; it had been part of the Indian culture for thousands of years,' he said. 'We do it all the

115

time, usually without being aware of it. You don't consider something a drug when it's the norm of your culture. It's just something you take.' Some of the older, legal drugs, such as alcohol and tobacco, are widely accepted, even though they probably do more harm than marijuana, possession of which is punishable by years in jail. The most dangerous drugs of all, amphetamines and barbiturates, are sometimes dispensed quite freely by doctors, and that is accepted. When we want to keep children and old people quiet, tranquillizers are accepted. It is time we viewed such practices more objectively.

'In the giving and taking of drugs,' write Dr Lennard and his colleagues, 'one pays for what one gets.' Whether the drugs are used for kicks, for self-enlightenment, for therapy, to sleep, to wake up or to control others, there is always a price to pay. Unforunately, one can seldom see the price-tag.

When Sigmund Freud first tried out cocaine on himself, while looking for possible medical uses for it, he became wildly enthusiastic. Calling the drug 'magical', he sent some to his fiancée, 'to make her strong and give her cheeks a red colour'. He wrote to her that a small dose of cocaine, which he took while feeling depressed, 'lifted me to the heights in a wonderful fashion'. He pressed the drug on his friends and colleagues, both for themselves and their patients, and he gave it to his sisters; in short, as his biographer, Ernest Jones, points out, 'he was rapidly becoming a public menace'. Little by little, the price became apparent. One friend developed a severe cocaine addiction and delirium tremens, which hastened his death. A patient died from an overdose. Soon Freud was attacked on all sides for having introduced the Western world to 'the third scourge of humanity' (after morphine and alcohol). He stopped using it, and even in his old age, while suffering so intensely from cancer that he saw his world as 'a little island of pain floating on a sea of indifference', he refused to take any drug whatsoever, relenting only occasionally to swallow some aspirin. 'I prefer to think in torment than not to be able to think clearly,' he declared. When the pain became totally unbearable, he saw no point in living further and asked his doctor to put an end to the torture. The doctor complied, giving him a small dose of morphine, which kept him unconscious until he died one day later. To the end, writes Jones, 'there was no emotionalism or self-pity, only reality'.

Despite the enormous increase in drug abuse in recent years, there are some signs that the epidemic may soon begin to recede. Those who are bent on destroying themselves or punishing their parents will always find a way. But other young people are becoming more selective in their search for kicks. Many experienced drug-users are giving up drugs for meditation, while the reverse is hardly ever true. Those who switch to meditation do so not for moral reasons, but simply because they like it better. Considering how few persons are really helped by drugs and how many are hurt, it is very fortunate that the kicks are now available without the chemical.

6 Changing the baby's brain: can intelligence, emotionality and sex be changed at will?

Nothing is left to chance in Aldous Huxley's *Brave New World*. Babies are born out of bottles ('decanted') in the state hatcheries where all human ova are stored, inspected and fertilized. As the bottles travel down conveyor belts, the caste system begins. The embryos that will become sewage workers are deliberately deprived of oxygen, to stunt their growth and turn them into Epsilon Semi-Morons. Those destined to become Alphas (the intellectuals and managers who rule the world) receive large quantities of oxygen and a variety of enriching substances. Other castes are physically and chemically prepared for specialized jobs such as repairing rockets in mid-air (the bottles are rotated to improve their sense of balance) or working in the tropics (a matter of heat-conditioning). At a certain point on the conveyor belt, a shot of male sex hormones makes two-thirds of all the female embryos infertile. And from birth on, all infants are conditioned to *like* their status. Their earliest experiences, are controlled with extreme care, to be further reinforced by repeated suggestions during their sleep. In this way, the state produces exactly the kind and number of people it needs.

Huxley, so prophetic in other ways, was wrong in one respect — it has not taken men six centuries to achieve such control over developing brains. Even now, only forty years later, *Brave New World* is nearly here, at least for laboratory animals. So much has been learned about critical periods in brain develop-

118

ment and the effects of early experience that men are beginning to shape in various ways the brains of rats, mice, salamanders and other creatures. At the same time, scientists have begun to turn their attention to the human infant. They are discovering how heredity, nutrition and experience work together to produce different castes of children in today's society. As yet they have little or no access to embryonic human brains, but with the development of test-tube babies that may not be far away.

Ever since Freud it has been known that a human being's character is formed by the experiences he has had before the age of five. Intelligence, however, was supposed to be fixed by heredity. There was no evidence that early experiences could in any way change the anatomy or chemistry of the brain.

The man most responsible for proving that such changes do in fact occur is Professor David Krech, a psychologist at the University of California at Berkeley. He was spending a year at the University of Oslo in 1950 when he ran into a Berkeley colleague whom he hardly knew, Professor Melvin Calvin, a chemist who later became a Nobel laureate. Far away from home, the two men suddenly found much to talk about, and Dr Krech told Dr Calvin how dissatisfied he was with current methods of studying the brain. Instead of cutting out parts of the brain to find out what abilities were lost as a result, he wanted to study how the brain functioned normally. Why not investigate how the brain's chemistry changed during different kinds of mental activity? Dr Calvin was delighted with this idea, which fitted his views about the power of chemistry, and they agreed to join forces when Dr Krech returned home.

In 1952, Dr Calvin introduced Dr Krech to Dr Edward Bennett, an associate of his and a biochemist. Together with Dr Bennett and Dr Mark Rosenzweig, a biological psychologist who had become interested in the transmission of nerve impulses, Dr Krech set out to study the relation between mental activity – particularly memory and learning – and the quantity of certain enzymes in the brains of rats.

Their reasoning went like this: mental activity must involve a flow of electrical impulses from neuron to neuron; this in turn requires both a chemical transmitter, such as acetylcholine, and an enzyme to break it up after it has done its job, such as acetylcholinesterase. The three researchers guessed that a greater mental activity would involve a greater supply of both chemicals, but that while the transmitter would be used up, the enzyme would persist. Therefore, mental activity might be accompanied by an increase in brain enzymes. This is what they set out to test. At first they studied how rats with different amounts of enzymes in their brains performed on different problems. Then, in 1959, they decided to try the reverse – to see whether different kinds of performance would result in different amounts of brain enzymes.

To do this they needed two equal groups of animals, one using its brains while the other sat in idleness. They also wanted animals that had had little previous experience. And so the University of California opened its first rat 'nursery school': a spacious, multi-level cage filled with ladders, slides, trapezes, blocks, cans, wheels, brushes and other toys, in which a dozen baby rats could find plenty of challenges. Meanwhile, their brothers and sisters remained cooped up either in 'standard' laboratory accommodations – small, barren, wire-mesh cages housing three animals – or, far worse, in 'impoverished' cages, where they lived alone – miniature San Quentins with three solid walls, dim lights and no noise. The differential treatment began when the rats were taken from their mothers at weaning (about twenty-five days after birth). They were kept in the three different conditions for eighty days. At 105 days after birth, all were decapitated, and their brains were instantly dissected, weighed and frozen by technicians.

The experiment had been going nicely for a couple of years, with just the right kind of evidence piling up – the nursery-school rats had 2 per cent more acetylcholinesterase in their brains than the others – when suddenly the researchers discovered something so revolutionary they could hardly believe it:

the cortex – the 'thinking' part of the brain – of the nursery-school rats weighed 4 per cent more than the cortex of the other rats' brains.

'We had inherited from our predecessors the dogma of absolute stability of brain weight,' recalled Dr Rosenzweig. Long ago, some anatomists had claimed that the brain grew through intellectual activity. This had led scientists to compare the size of different persons' brains at autopsy, but they only succeeded in proving that brain size was no guide to intelligence, for idiots sometimes had larger brains than geniuses. By the beginning of the twentieth century, the search for brain changes that could be attributed to experience had been abandoned. Even the Berkeley team did not expect to find more than the subtlest chemical changes in the brain as a result of learning; grosser effects, such as weight changes, seemed beyond the realm of possibility, and were not included in the experiment. 'Fortunately,' said Dr Rosenzweig, 'we had to record the weights of our brain samples in order to measure chemical activity per unit of tissue weight. After about two years of contemplating the chemical effects, it finally dawned on us that the weights of the brain samples also changed.'

At first glance, the Berkeley rats' brains seemed unaltered by their stay in the nursery school. However, the researchers had cut up the brains into various sections and weighed each separately. A little elementary arithmetic showed that the cortex of the impoverished rats was smaller than that of the nursery-school graduates. Evidently, the experience of playing with a wide variety of toys for eighty days had impelled the rats' cortex to grow.

This fact spurred the team to renewed activity. They had to find out what the heavier cortex was filling itself out with. Soon a neuroanatomist, Professor Marian Diamond, joined the team to look for the anatomical changes. The discoveries made by Dr Diamond and her lab proved perhaps most startling of all. Among the first things she noticed was an actual thickening of the rats' cortex, especially in the visual areas at the back of the

121

brain. (This later turned out to be true even in blinded rats.) There was also a 15 per cent increase in the number of glial cells, housekeeping cells that play a mysterious but important role in learning. The number of nerve cells, or neurons, had not increased (it is generally believed that neurons cannot reproduce after birth), but the cell bodies had become 15 per cent larger. The fibres of these neurons had also grown and proliferated, creating new neural branches with which to make connections with other cells. The entire quality of the cortex had changed.

Among mammals, intelligence always corresponds to the size and complexity of the cerebral cortex. In rats the cortex is smooth and comparatively underdeveloped. Going up the evolutionary ladder, the cortex of dogs begins to show some convolutions, thus packing more cortex into the available space. In monkeys the cortex is further expanded and convoluted, and in man is so highly developed that it overshadows all other parts of the brain. If an animal's cortex became enlarged through experience, then would its intelligence also increase? This proved very difficult to measure, because animals that score high on one kind of test and thus appear more intelligent sometimes do poorly on another, and vice versa. It all depends on the abilities one chooses to test. But, clearly, some strains of animals can be bred for skills on specific tests.

Years before, as a graduate student at Berkeley, Dr Krech had watched the psychologist Robert Tryon demonstrate how differently two strains of rats behaved in a maze. Professor Tryon had bred these strains selectively for generations. The rats whose ancestors had been selected for 'maze-dullness' would enter a maze, hit a dead-end, and then make mistake after mistake, day after day, never seeming to learn their way, while it took those of the 'maze-bright' strain only a few tries to scoot right through. 'What I was seeing, of course, was one of psychology's classic experiments,' Dr Krech said, 'indeed *the* experiment which established behaviour genetics as an experimental science.' It was bound to shake anyone's belief in the prime importance of the environment as opposed to heredity. But now Dr Krech was ready for a new experiment. Descendants of the two strains of rats – among the prize possessions of the psychology department at Berkeley – were still available, and even though the selection process had stopped forty years earlier, the brains of the two strains still differed. They had different amounts of enzymes in their brains, and different ratios of cortex to sub-cortex. Other rat strains could also be shown to differ genetically, both in ability to learn certain skills and in brain chemistry. The next question was to what extent different environments could change these hereditary traits.

Thirty rats that were genetically gifted at learning maze problems were placed in impoverished cages, while less gifted rats were placed in the enriched environment. This virtually wiped out the strain differences between their brains. On the other hand, the opposite treatment – giving gifted rats the benefits of enriched conditions while the others stayed in impoverished cages – actually doubled the difference between them.

'We can now undo the effects of generations of breeding,' declared Dr Krech. 'Heredity is not enough. All the advantages of inheriting a good brain can be lost if you don't have the right psychological environment in which to develop it.' Simply by changing their early environments, he could change the anatomy and chemistry of the brains of rats that were born inferior (or at least less talented at certain tasks), making them equal to their former superiors.

Among the rats' toughest tasks was learning that rules can change – an important aspect of intelligence. The test for this was called a 'reversal discrimination' problem. As soon as the animals learned to choose the darker of two alleys for a food reward, the opposite alley began to be rewarded. A number of rats learned the principle of the thing rapidly. They would try one alley, discover the rule of the day, then go on with hardly an error. But others never learned. On this 'IQ' test, the evidence was absolutely clear: the gifted rats performed far better than the others at all times, except when they, alone, had been deprived of stimulation in infancy. When the duller rats were sent to the nursery school and the brights kept in isolated cages, the brights deteriorated so much that they made an average of thirty-two mistakes, while the dulls developed sufficiently to make only twenty-one.

If one wants to make an animal more intelligent, concluded Dr Krech after a long series of experiments, love is not enough; physical exercise is not enough; visual stimulation is neither necessary nor sufficient; the presence of other young animals is not enough; and deliberate teaching helps, but not much. The only experience that really stretches a rat's brain is the opportunity to explore a large number of different objects, or a large variety of mazes. According to Dr Krech, this is a species-specific requirement, since rats need to have good 'space-brains'. Human beings have different requirements, he believes, mostly connected with language, although he cannot prove it. However, he did prove that by manipulating the environment of the young, one can truly create a 'lame brain'. Or one can create a better brain and a cleverer animal, at will.

By now Dr Krech has retired from the Berkeley team to do research on a new topic: intra-uterine environments. Together with a number of scientists who keep pushing back the age of their research subjects, he suspects that the environment before birth is a key factor in determining individual differences in intelligence, brain structure and other traits.

Meanwhile, the other members of the team are continuing to study the effects of enriched environments on the brains of rats, mice and gerbils at various times after birth. They have found that cortical changes are easier to produce than they had originally supposed: two hours a day of experience in the enriched cages seem to change the brains of rats just as much as keeping them there all day long. Furthermore, the animals don't have to be put into the nursery school right after weaning – brain changes are possible at any age. Since the differences between the animals' performances tend to disappear after repeated testing, the team does not believe that the effects of early environment are irreversible.

However, even if it isn't true that you can't teach an old brain new tricks, it does take very much longer. When the team gave middle-aged rats the chance to play with and explore all the toys in the nursery school, for instance, the animals' cortex/subcortex ratio increased considerably after ninety days. The same increase could be achieved in adolescent rats after only thirty days, however. And neither group gained as much from the experience as did animals that went into the nursery school in earliest infancy, with their mothers, even before they were weaned.

These experiments tend to support the psychologist Benjamin Bloom's theory that the easiest time to make a profound change in a child's intelligence is while that intelligence is growing most rapidly, before the age of four. Dr Bloom, a professor of education at the University of Chicago, analysed over a thousand longitudinal studies of growth and noted that there is a specific growth curve for each human characteristic. Half a child's eventual height, for instance, is reached by the age of two-and-a-half. By the age of four, his IQ becomes so stable that it is a fairly accurate indicator of his intelligence and maturity. Dr Bloom then formulated a general rule: the environment will have maximum impact on a specific trait during that trait's period of most rapid growth. As time goes by, more and more powerful forces are required to produce a given amount of change, if it can be produced at all. This rule now appears to apply equally well to the structure of the brain, since brain changes can be brought about most easily and dramatically shortly after birth, at a time when the brain is growing at top speed.

The Berkeley group also found that, whatever the rats' ages, their brains did not change if they were alone in the nursery school. Dr Rosenzweig attributes this to the fact that solitary rats don't pay much attention to their surroundings, but tend to rest or to groom themselves. To make their brains grow, he had to 'con' them into getting involved with their playthings. If a rat was hungry, for example, Dr Rosenzweig could stimulate it by placing food at various spots inside or on top of the toys, thus forcing it to 'play'. Solitary rats could also be stimulated by moderate doses of excitant drugs, which made them so active that they interacted with everything around them. Or else they could be stimulated by novelty: just like children, rats, even those that live in groups, become bored with their toys if they have them too long.

If new puzzles and challenges can make the cortex grow, *more* new puzzles and challenges every day make it grow more rapidly, judging from some experiments by a young Argentinian couple, Pedro and Vesna Ferchmin, who unwittingly improved on the Berkeley team's methods. The Ferchmins had read about the team's work and wanted to reproduce it in Argentina, but they did not know exactly how. Forced to devise their own procedures, they invented a supercharged environment so powerful that it produced many of the brain changes normally seen after thirty days in the short space of four days.

Surely no rat could get bored in the Ferchmin régime, which the young researchers have now introduced to Berkeley. The animals are moved three times a day, first from a standard laboratory cage to a larger one much like the original Berkeley rat nursery school, then to an oversize, five-foot-high cage with a most intricate and imaginative assortment of toys. The rats' ingenuity is sharply challenged by such problems as how to reach the top shelf on one side of the cage, for instance, when there is no direct access to it. They have to figure out a roundabout route across a series of nesting houses perched on vertical rods, across some diagonal chains and over some boxes. The problems keep changing, as the layout of the cage is completely altered every day.

In addition, as in any well-run nursery school, the rats in the Ferchmin cage have teachers. Four older animals, whom the Ferchmins call 'masters', serve as experienced models for baby rats to imitate when they are introduced into the cage. This appears to accelerate their learning tremendously. Certainly the rats in the Ferchmin cage are more active than any others, and their brains also change more rapidly.

The best explanation of why rats, like children, 'learn by doing' comes from some recent work by scientists at MIT. The key to it is feedback – the information that the brain receives both about its own efforts and about their results. An animal cannot learn a new motor skill just by looking, because this involves no feedback. It must try out certain movements, and it must try them out *voluntarily*.

This enormous difference between voluntary and passive movement is an exciting concept. A person who looks up at something voluntarily is well aware that the rest of the room has not moved, even though his angle of vision has changed. Yet if his eyeballs are moved by an outside force, or even by his own fingers, his field of vision seems to jump. This shows that something very central is changed by intention. His brain sends out signals to prepare him for the consequences of his voluntary acts. The same holds true for animals, as scientists in Germany and California have shown. Professor Roger Sperry, of the California Institute of Technology, calls this internal signal a 'corollary discharge', since it closely follows the brain's more direct command to muscles to move. And at MIT, the psychologists Richard Held and Alan Hein have produced evidence that corollary discharges are essential to adaptation, especially in newborns. Without such signals, one could not learn to cope with one's environment.

In Dr Held's and Dr Hein's laboratory, I tried on some goggles that grossly distorted the room and made my hands seem far away from where I expected them to be. The goggles contained prisms, I was told; all objects appeared to be tilted dizzyingly, and as I tried to move, I found it very difficult to orient myself. Several pairs of volunteers had been tested with the goggles by Professor Held. One goggled member of each pair stood on a sort of cart, almost at floor level, while the other person wheeled him about, so that both covered exactly the same territory. At the end of an hour, the volunteers who had done the pushing had adapted to their goggles so completely that they could reach any object with ease and no longer saw any distortion. It was only when they removed the goggles that the room appeared lopsided to them. Clearly a change had taken place in their brains. However, their partners had learned nothing from the experience. They still misjudged all distances with the goggles on, but returned to normal as soon as the goggles were removed.

Before brains can be shaped through feedback, then, there must be a sort of 'feedforward' to compare it with. This is why infants need to move their hands so much, why babies want to grab hold of everything, why toddlers must experiment with sounds before they can speak. Voluntary acts are essential to brain development. But they can be induced, as the Berkeley team found out, by making the environment sufficiently interesting or challenging.

Everything the newborn does or fails to do shapes its brain, sometimes irreversibly. For in all animals, and presumably man, there are critical periods of development, during which certain things *must* happen or it will be too late.

It takes only four days to kill off the marvellous 'feature detectors' in the brains of kittens, for instance. These 'feature detectors' are cells in the visual cortex that specialize in identifying patterns and shapes. If a kitten's eye is kept closed for four days during the critical period (which for cats is the fourth week of life, according to recent work by David Hubel and Thorsten Wiesel of Harvard), it loses its connections to the cortex, so that the other eye becomes permanently dominant. If both eyes are kept covered for a few weeks, the cat will be functionally blind. The loss can also be quite subtle: Colin Blakemore of the Physiological Laboratory in Cambridge, England, has shown that when kittens grow up in a world where they see only vertical lines, they become relatively blind to horizontal lines, and vice versa. In such cases, only certain kinds of 'feature detectors' can be found in the kitten's visual cortex –

those that were stimulated by either vertical or horizontal lines in early life. It is an amazingly specific demonstration of the power of the environment.

An even more dramatic and irrevocable change occurs in the behaviour of ducklings. It is a once-in-a-lifetime event, limited to a short period during their first twenty-four hours out of the egg. During that time, the duckling is uniquely impressionable, and whatever it sees most conspicuously – usually the shape of its mother – becomes permanently etched into its brain. From then on, the duck will follow this shape slavishly. The ethnologist Konrad Lorenz called this phenomenon 'imprinting'. There are memorable films of Lorenz striding along, followed by a line of ducklings that saw only him during their critical period, and as a result treated him as if he were their mother. The ducklings on which he was imprinted felt a compulsion to follow him. They would go to any lengths, and brave any danger, just to be with him. Since Dr Lorenz's pioneering experiments other researchers have imprinted chicks and ducklings with toys, boxes and flashing lights, as well as human beings. They have found that the chicks and ducks will follow all these objects with the same unquestioning allegiance. If a chick hatches exceptionally late it may miss the critical period. In that case, nothing will ever be imprinted on it, and its brain will contain less newly made RNA and protein than the brains of chicks that have learned, through imprinting, who their 'mother' is.

Most of what is known about critical periods in the development of the human brain is tragic. At certain stages during the first three months of pregnancy, for instance, the German measles virus can irreparably damage the foetus's brain, though later in pregnancy it may do no harm. The brains of millions of babies are being stunted every day, as a result of poor nutrition at critical times. It has become absolutely clear, from studies by paediatricians such as Herbert Birch, of the Albert Einstein College of Medicine, and Myron Winick, of the Institute of Human Nutrition at Columbia University, that low-protein

E

diets damage children's brains, and that if this occurs before six months of age the damage may be irreversible.

'There is no recovery in organs where cell division has already stopped,' said Dr Winick. 'The brain never gets another chance.' He found that Chilean children who had been under nourished as infants were still mentally retarded five years later. Only those whose poor diets started at a later age recovered after prolonged rehabilitation.

High-protein diets seem to be essential during two particularly sensitive periods, judging from studies on the brains of rats: during the second half of the mother's pregnancy, when the central nervous system is developing rapidly and the brain's neurons are dividing at top speed, and during the first six months of life, when the brain's glial cells are increasing most rapidly. 'Prenatal malnutrition results in a 15 per cent reduction in cell number at birth,' Dr Winick said. 'Postnatal malnutrition results in a reduction of similar magnitude by weaning.' Each of these represents severe deprivation. However, when an animal is undernourished during both of these critical periods, he suffers a *60 per cent reduction* in the number of his brain cells by the time he is weaned.

This 'double deprivation' is most likely to occur when a child is born prematurely. This is why the late Dr Birch urged a drive to provide planned nutritional supplements for high-risk mothers. Among poor families, and especially poor black families, nearly a quarter of all babies are born prematurely, largely because the mother is not getting proper nourishment during her pregnancy. These babies are then prime candidates for later intellectual deficiency. 'The long-term consequences of these early insults are greatest when the chronic circumstances in which the child grows . . . are substandard,' said Dr Birch. He also advocated an aggressive programme of parent education with regard to nutrition.

The babies who survived such horrors as the famines of Bangladesh, Afghanistan and Biafra may thus be mentally crippled for life. Around the world, and especially in under-

130

developed countries, millions of children are regularly deprived of sufficient proteins to keep their brains growing at a normal rate, and in times of crisis entire generations of infants are condemned to brain damage. Yet inexpensive proteins are now available from many sources. No wonder that the president of the American Orthopsychiatric Association, Dr Benjamin Pasamanick, recently called the people of the United States 'a cheap, murderous lot' because they recognize the problem of hunger and do nothing about it. It is a form of atrocity by omission.

But the human body is a marvellous instrument. Despite their vulnerability, newborns sometimes show enormous resilience, functioning well despite injuries that would be catastrophic to an adult. This is because the brain can mend itself best while it is growing most rapidly. It seems to compensate for the loss of one structure by letting another one expand and take over. There are critical periods for that, too. Like all critical periods, they exist because different areas of the brain develop at different rates.

First comes the inner core, the brain stem, which controls arousal and consciousness. The cerebellum, which controls physical balance, and the cerebral cortex, which swells to such enormous bulk in man, mature much later, under a complicated timetable. Many scientists now agree with the Russian physiologist P. K. Anokhin, who attributed this order to the demands of natural selection: the parts of the brain that are most essential to the newborn's survival mature first. Within this general framework, however, little is yet known, since the science of growth is itself still in infancy.

At the National Institute of Mental Health in Bethesda, Maryland, a young neuropsychologist, Dr Patricia Goldman, has been studying the brain's power of self-repair. She was intrigued by a number of reversals in the development of brain-injured animals. Some baby monkeys that had seemed most severely handicapped after brain surgery eventually caught up with and surpassed the performance of others that had seemed least troubled. After a series of experiments Dr Goldman developed a theory of 'differential commitment'. Only tissue that is highly immature and still uncommitted to a particular course of development can take on new functions, she believes (assuming that it is functionally related to the injured part). In adults, all pathways remaining after a brain injury would presumably be 'fixed', so that it would be too late for anatomical reorganization. 'The basic question,' she said, 'is whether what's left in the brain is sufficiently immature.'

When more is known about the mosaic of differential maturation in various regions of the brain, it may be possible to shape the brains of infants, or even foetuses, quite effectively, much as Huxley foresaw in *Brave New World*.

Also as in *Brave New World* – but only for rats – it is already possible to alter sex during a critical period right after birth by an injection of hormones that act on the infant rat's brain. If one were dealing with human beings, the injections would have to take place before birth, just as Huxley imagined. But rats are born deaf and blind and still relatively close to the foetal state, and for a brief period of life their sex can be changed.

Sex is set in the brain, the British physiologist Geoffrey Harris of the Institute of Psychology demonstrated in 1965. It depends on specific events in the brain at various stages before and immediately after birth. And despite the story of Adam and Eve, in the beginning, all brains are female.

'It is a struggle to become a male,' commented Dr Seymour Levine, a psychiatrist now at Stanford University who worked with Dr Harris. 'It is an additive process.' The proper male hormones must act upon the brain at the proper time for the brain to set patterns of maleness throughout the central nervous system. If the brain is not triggered in time, the foetus remains female. Even after birth, depriving a newborn male rat's brain of male hormones for the first twenty-four hours of life will cause him to become functionally female. He will still have male organs, but he will develop a regular hormonal cycle, as if preparing for ovulation and menstruation. Similarly, female rats can be turned into pseudo-males by a single injection of male hormone right after birth. The hormone apparently acts on their hypothalamus. From then on, they never ovulate and never show any female patterns of sexual receptivity. If treated with more male hormones later in life, they even attempt to mount other females and go through the motions of copulation, as if they were males.

Obviously, knowledge of an animal's critical periods gives one enormous power to change its whole course of development. Scientists are just beginning to discover the relevant timetables – the critical periods, both before and after birth, for sex, intelligence, emotionality and dozens of other traits. Some of their interventions may prove extremely valuable. And since timing is such a powerful factor, they may look deceptively mild.

'One of the most striking facts is that what appear to be *minimal* changes in the early environment have proved to have profound effects on the subsequent performance of the developing organism,' declared Dr Levine. In 1956 he had set out to prove some aspects of 'what we took to be Freudian theory at the time – the long-term effects of infantile trauma.' He separated some newborn rats into three groups. One group received electric shocks for three minutes a day; the rats in the second group were also taken from their mothers and placed in a different cage for three minutes a day, but were given no electric shocks; the third group was left alone, to serve as a control. 'Our assumption was that since it would be having the best of all possible worlds – living with a warm, nutrient, moist mother, not being disturbed, and having all the comforts of life – it [the third group] would essentially not be affected in any way', Dr Levine explained. 'We assumed the outcome would be basically the same as in our handled but non-shocked group, and that only the group given shock trauma would turn out to be different. Well, the rest of it is history! To our surprise, we found out that there were very profound effects from *lack* of stimulation, and that not doing anything at all to the rats was worst of all.'

Dr Levine discovered that *any* kind of early experience – handling, or even more traumatic things such as electric shocks or vigorous shaking – seemed to make the animals more emotionally stable. As adults, such rats were better able to learn, better able to cope with new environments, more curious and more likely to have appropriate responses in any given situation. In the laboratory, where the rats were kept in racks of cages, it was striking to see that all the handled animals occupied the front of their cages, while the non-handled ones huddled at the back. When food was put into their cages, the handled animals ate it right away; the non-handled rats still hadn't touched theirs fifteen minutes later. In an 'open field' test too, the animals that had been handled for a few days after birth showed more sense than the others. If they weren't hungry, they nearly always chose to explore the field; however, if they had been deprived of food, they quite reasonably made a beeline for whatever could be eaten. The non-handled rats were much less flexible: satiated or not, they never ventured into the field on first exposure, but always sought the security of the food. Dr Levine points out that although the non-handled rats did eventually get accustomed to such open fields and could not be distinguished from the handled rats, their basic predisposition did not change. If something new happened to them – for instance, if a loud bell was rung – the non-handled rats again froze in a corner, too frightened to move. 'Behaviour therapy can be used to reverse certain effects of early experience,' Dr Levine said, 'but this doesn't mean that a permanent or chronic reversal will be obtained over the whole spectrum of behaviour that is affected by early experience.'

In his experiments, the non-handled rats spent their first days of life in barren cages much like those of the Berkeley group's 'impoverished' rats. He does not view this as a state of deprivation, however, since in this case the animals were with their mothers, who kept licking them, biting them and picking them up. Instead, he speaks about the lack of novelty in their environment. The laboratory was soundproofed, evenly lighted and air-conditioned, and the baby rats never left their cages. This prevented them from developing much of a basis for matching one kind of novelty with another, he believes, so that 'each set of circumstances was seen as unique and . . . they were continually thrown by novel environments'. Having more things to habituate to, compare and match, the handled rats rapidly learned to generalize from one environment to the next.

'It's not intelligence, but better functioning,' Dr Levine concluded. He feels that early experience with novelty will produce animals that are emotionally stable enough to perform well. Of course, if they are over-aroused, as with too much electric shock, they will do poorly – there is an optimum level. 'I couldn't possibly give a good lecture unless I were a little anxious,' he said, 'but I would freeze and couldn't give the lecture at all if I were over-anxious.' Apparently, newborns need various kinds of stimulation to set their arousal threshold at the appropriate level. And within broad limits, any stimulation is better than none. 'I don't care how bright you are,' Dr Levine said, 'if you're frightened to death, you can't function.'

All the effects of early and varied experience – a higher cortex/subcortex ratio, greater intelligence, more curiosity, less fear – obviously reinforce each other. An animal that is less frightened will explore more, get more involved with his surroundings, and learn more. An animal that has learned more will have more flexibility and be less likely to freeze into inaction.

Early malnutrition also has a dual effect: a direct one on brain anatomy, and an indirect one on the animal's ability to learn, since it may rob him of the energy for much voluntary activity. In effect, this apathy restricts the animal's environment. However, the cycle can be broken at any place. Even with a low-protein diet, stimulation in infancy can be helpful. In some experiments with rats at Cornell University, researchers have found that early handling and a rich selection of toys to play with in an interesting environment can largely counteract the bad effects of malnutrition after birth.

A psychologist at the University of Connecticut, Dr Victor Denenberg, has discovered that he can change the level of violence of mice simply by giving them a different education, if he starts right after birth. Using a strain of mice known to be extremely aggressive – their young males were notorious for their constant fights – he removed half of one litter from a mouse mother on the day of birth and had these babies raised by a female rat. At twenty-one days of age the mice were placed in standard 'fighting-boxes', small boxes in which a barrier between two animals is suddenly lowered, leaving them face-to-face with a stranger. Against all expectations, the mice that had been raised by the rat mother refused to fight one another. Dr Denenberg, who had long been interested in the effects of early experience but had no idea what he would find in this case, was astounded that he could turn off the species-specific pattern of fighting in this way. To make sure that some chemical factor in the rat mother's milk was not responsible, he repeated the experiment with a group of mice nursed by their natural mother but otherwise raised by a rat 'aunt', who took over most of the mothering duties. This time some of the young males did fight, but the majority did not. Apparently the mere presence of a rat 'aunt' during this critical period in their lives had changed the mice sufficiently to cut down the episodes of aggression to less than half the usual number.

Slowly, then, we are beginning to learn how to make a superior brain. It is a matter of programming, of providing the most favourable environment for specific needs at various critical times both before and after birth. Of course the genes set limits beyond which one cannot go, but these are so broad that nobody ever reaches them, and they leave room for infinite variations according to circumstances. Man's intelligence, for instance, may vary up to 40 IQ points, depending on his environment, according to Professor Samuel Kirk of the University of

Arizona. More conservatively, Benjamin Bloom estimates that a child's environment is responsible for roughly 20 IQ points – still a formidable span, he points out; one that could mean the difference between life in an institution for the feeble-minded and a productive life in society, or between a professional career and an occupation at the semi-skilled or unskilled level. By the age of four, the direction is usually quite clear.

In some respects, the direction is clear even before birth. When pregnant rats were exposed to glaring lights, which terrified them, their fear made them produce hormones that feminized, or demasculinized, their male offspring. Later on these males failed to copulate with inviting females. Even though no drugs were used, their sex had been changed as if by hormones, simply by changing their mother's environment while she carried them.

This means that the reverse is also true: by deliberately altering an expectant mother's environment, we may learn to counteract accidents of nature and prevent harm to the unborn baby. For example, should a mother who is carrying a male foetus be badly frightened at a critical time during her pregnancy, an immediate dose of male hormones or their equivalent might prove helpful. The day may come when pregnant women will be monitored almost daily, to determine what critical period their baby is entering, and what specific programming would best suit it.

Prenatal programming of the brain could include chemical intervention – special foods, hormones, perhaps drugs if necessary; physical intervention, possibly along the lines of the 'decompression' treatments pioneered by a South African physician, Dr O. S. Heyns, which reduce pressure on the mother's womb and increase the amount of oxygen available to the foetus during the last ten days of pregnancy (the babies born after these treatments are said to be exceptionally intelligent and well developed); and psychological intervention, which may be the most difficult to develop. It is well known that babies born of mothers who live near airports or in the path of jet planes react differently to sound from other infants. The old wives' tales about maternal impressions – the stories about children marked forever by some event in their mothers' lives just before they were born – may yet turn out to have more than a grain of truth.

The period immediately after birth is probably the most promising. The baby is born with a huge head for his size, with a brain weighing one quarter of its adult weight, but during his first six months of life his brain weight will double. The glial cells will multiply, the neurons will branch out in a wealth of dendrites, and the little spines on the dendrites will sprout magically to receive connections from other cells. It is a time of explosive growth – and yet the human infant has the longest period of helplessness of any animal. His cortex takes longer to mature than any other creature's. Just because his cortex is so big and takes so long to develop, the environment has ample time and opportunities to shape it. We are only beginning to discover how it does so. Only in recent years have scientists begun to study and rate home environments, for instance – to clock what parents do to infants, to classify the kinds of interactions that take place, to record the language that is spoken.

Within a few decades, it should be in our power – as it is only partly today – to produce the kinds of brains we want. We will know how nutrition, chemistry, activity, environmental variety and other factors interact to shape the baby's brain. We will know how to produce Alphas or Betas, as well as Epsilon Semi-Morons. It will be simply a matter of choice.

7 Which half of your brain is dominant: and can you change it?

Linked together like Siamese twins right down the middle of our brains, two very different persons inhabit our heads. One of them is verbal, analytical, dominant. The other is artistic but mute, and still almost totally mysterious.

These are the left and right hemispheres of our brains, the twin shells that cover the central brain stem. In normal people, they are connected by millions of nerve fibres which form a thick cable called the corpus callosum. If this cable is cut, as must be done in certain cases of severe epilepsy, a curious set of circumstances occurs. The left side of the brain no longer knows what the right side is doing, yet the speaking half of the patient, controlled by the left hemisphere, still insists on finding excuses for whatever the mute half has done, and still operates under the illusion that they are one person.

As a result of these extraordinary findings of the past decade, brain scientists have begun to wonder whether our normal feeling of being just one person is also an illusion, even though our brains remain whole. Are the two halves of our brains integrated into a single soul? Is one hemisphere always dominant over the other? Or do the two persons in our brains take turns at directing our activities and thoughts?

Theologians are not alone in watching this research with fascination – and some misgivings. It has aroused the interest of many others who are concerned with human identity. As they soon realize, all roads lead to the psychobiologist Roger Sperry,

139

who has the gift of making – or provoking – important discoveries.

Professor Sperry was already famous before he began studying people and animals whose brains had been split in two. In a series of elegant experiments, he had shown that there exists a very precise chemical coding system during brain growth that allows specific nerve cells – for example, those concerned with vision – to find their way through a tangle of other nerve fibres, even when obstacles are placed in their path, and somehow connect with the appropriate cells so as to reach specific terminals in the visual cortex. Next he began to study visual perception and memory. He wanted to find out what happened when an animal learned certain discriminations that involved the visual cortex – when it learned, for instance, to push a panel marked with a circle rather than a square. Where in its brain was that knowledge stored?

He put the question to a young graduate student, suggesting that he should investigate how cats that have learned a new skill with only one eye and one hemisphere transfer this information to the other eye. The student, Ronald Myers (now chief of the Laboratory of Perinatal Physiology at the National Institute of Neurological Diseases and Stroke), worked with this idea for the next six years. First he developed a method of cutting through the cats' optic chiasm (the point at which the optic nerves meet and cross) so as to sever the nerve fibres that normally cross from left eye to right hemisphere and vice versa, sparing only those that connect with the same side of the brain. Despite the surgery, the cats saw quite well. Myers then placed a patch over one of their eyes and trained the one-eyed creatures to distinguish between a circle and a square, knowing that the information they acquired would go to only one hemisphere. When he switched their eye patches to cover their trained eyes, however, the cats performed just as well as before. Their memory of this skill was intact. This meant either that the knowledge was stored in the central brain stem, well below the twin hemispheres, or that the knowledge acquired by one hemisphere had somehow been transmitted to the other.

'Obviously the corpus callosum was the next thing to test,' says Dr Myers. 'But from the available evidence, cutting it would have no effect. If the surgery is properly done, the animals are up the next day and you see nothing.' By all outward appearances, a split-brained cat or monkey is perfectly normal: it can run, eat, mate, solve problems as if nothing had happened to it. When surgeons first split the brain of a human being in the 1930s (to remove a tumour deep in the brain), they did so with much trepidation, expecting a terrible change in their patient, a total deterioration of his psyche. To their amazement, they saw no change at all. The corpus callosum seemed to serve no purpose, despite its large size (it is about $3\frac{1}{2}$ inches long and a quarter of an inch thick in humans). 'What is the function of the corpus callosum?' professors would ask their students in the 1940s; as no one knew, they replied facetiously, 'It transmits epileptic seizures from one hemisphere to the other.' As recently as 1951, the well-known Harvard neuropsychologist Karl Lashley saw only one other use for it: 'To keep the hemispheres from sagging.'

Nevertheless, Dr Myers proceeded with the next step in the research plan. After cutting through the cats' optic chiasm, he split their corpus callosum as well, separating their left and right hemispheres. Then he trained them as before, with one eye covered. When he removed the cover from this eye and placed it over the other eye, however, there was a dramatic change: the cats reacted as if they had never seen the patterns before. They took just as long to learn the difference between a circle and a square with the second eye as they had with the first. Dr Myers was elated, and the question was finally settled: it was the corpus callosum that transmitted memories and learning from one hemisphere to the other. The thick band of fibres stood revealed at the sole means of communication between the two halves of the cerebral cortex. Without it, cats could be trained quite separately with each eye. When Dr Myers tried teaching

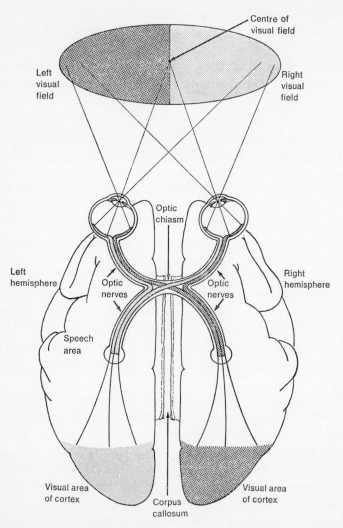

Visual Input to the Bisected Brain
From 'The Split Brain in Man' by Michael S. Gazzaniga. Copyright
© 1967 by Scientific American, Inc. All rights reserved.

142

some split-brained cats to select the circle with their left eye and the square with their right, he found that they learned this without the slightest evidence of conflict. They would act in opposite ways, according to which eye was open – as if they had two entirely separate brains.

In animals, a split brain may prove relatively unimportant. After all, both hemispheres are enclosed in a single head, attached to a single body, and normally exposed to identical experiences. Furthermore, the left and right halves of their brains do exactly the same job. But this is not the case for human beings.

Alone among the mammals, man has developed different uses for each half of his brain. This asymmetry, which we all recognize when we say whether we're right- or left-handed, is the glorious mechanism through which man is enabled to speak. It is what separates us from the apes. There are various theories about how it developed and whether it is present right from birth, but it is quite clear that by the time a child reaches the age of ten, one hemisphere – usually the left – has taken over the task of language.

For simpler operations, such as receiving sensations from one's hand or ordering movements to one's foot, the human brain remains generally symmetrical. The nerve impulses that carry messages from one side of the body travel up the spinal column and cross over into the opposite side of the brain, there to form a sort of mirror image of the parts they represent. The nerve connections involved are set at birth in an incredibly precise fashion that allows the brain to know instantly where certain sensations come from and where to aim specific instructions.

When tasks become more complex, however, this mirror-like representation is abandoned. Then the association areas of the brain come into play and each one develops in its own way, according to experience. Since we have only one mouth (unlike the dolphin, which has separate phonation mechanisms on the right and left sides of its body), there is no need for right and

143

left speech centres in the brain. On the contrary, these might conflict with each other and compete for control of the speech mechanism. In most adults, therefore, the speech centres are limited to one side of the brain, usually the left, though about 15 per cent of left-handers and perhaps 2 per cent of right-handers have speech on both sides.

Being left-handed – an inherited trait – generally means that the two sides of one's brain have not become as fully specialized as among right-handers. The 10 per cent of the population who are left-handed in childhood tend to be ambidextrous, and according to some research by the University of Pennsylvania's Dr Jerre Levy they often score much lower on tests of perceptual or motor ability. Furthermore, there are two kinds of left-handers: those whose language is controlled by the right hemisphere (less than half the total), and those in whom the left hemisphere controls speech, just as in right-handers.

This makes the left side of the brain largely dominant for language in human beings – a near-monopoly that was recognized in the nineteenth century, when surgeons examined the brains of people who had lost the power of speech and found severe damage on the left side. Why this should be so pre-ordained is not clear. The left hemisphere tends to become dominant in other ways as well. For example, it controls the right hand, which does most of man's skilled work with tools.

Around the age of one, the psychologist Jerome Bruner has observed, babies suddenly master what he calls 'the two-handed obstacle box', a simple puzzle developed by the Center for Cognitive Studies at Harvard to study how babies learn the value of two-handedness. The baby will push and hold a transparent cover with one hand, for the first time, while the other hand reaches inside the box for a toy, even though nobody has taught him this skill. To Dr Bruner this seems extraordinary, for it shows that the baby has learned to distinguish between two kinds of grip – the power, or 'holding', grip, which stabilizes an object, usually with the left hand, and the precision, or 'operating', grip, which does the work, usually with the right. Mon-

144

keys and apes also develop a precision grip, Dr Bruner told me, but only in man, with his asymmetry, does the power grip migrate to the left hand while the precision grip migrates to the right. This is the beginning of a long road leading to the distinctively human use of tools and toolmaking.

If the left hemisphere does all this, why do we need a right hemisphere? Experiments with split-brained cats and monkeys could not shed much light on the differing specialities of man's two hemispheres. The study of the two personalities in our brain did not really begin until 1961, when Dr Sperry became interested in a forty-eight-year-old veteran whose head had been hit by bomb fragments during the Second World War.

A few years after his injury, W.J. had begun to have epileptic fits; these became so frequent and so severe that nothing could control them. He would fall down, unconscious and foaming at the mouth, often hurting himself as he fell. For more than five years, doctors at the White Memorial Medical Center in Los Angeles tried every conceivable remedy, without success. Finally Dr Philip Vogel and Dr Joseph Bogen cut through his corpus callosum, and the seizures stopped, as if by magic. There was a difficult period of recovery, during which W.J., a man of above average intelligence, could not speak, but within a month he announced that he felt better than he had in years. He appeared unchanged in personality and perfectly normal.

Meanwhile, Dr Sperry had interested a graduate student, Michael Gazzaniga, in performing a series of tests on W.J., together with himself and Dr Bogen. Gazzaniga soon discovered some extremely odd things about his subject. To begin with, W.J. could carry out verbal commands ('raise your hand', or 'bend your knee') only with the right side of his body. He could not respond with his left side. Evidently the right hemisphere, which controls the left limbs, did not understand that kind of language. When W.J. was blindfolded, he couldn't even tell what part of his body was touched, if it happened to be on the left side.

In fact, as the tests proceeded, it became increasingly difficult to think of W.J. as a single person. His left hand kept doing things that his right hand deplored, if it was aware of them at all. Sometimes he would try to pull his pants down with one hand, while pulling them up with the other. Once he threatened his wife with his left hand while his right hand tried to come to his wife's rescue and bring the belligerent hand under control. Dr Gazzaniga, now a professor of psychology at the State University of New York at Stony Brook, recalls that he was walking with W.J. in the patient's back yard when W.J. picked up an axe with his left hand. Alarmed, Dr Gazzaniga discreetly left the scene. 'It was entirely likely that the more aggressive right hemisphere might be in control,' he explains. And since he couldn't communicate with it, he didn't want to be the victim in a test case of 'which half-brain does society punish or execute'.

Only the left half-brain could speak. The right one remained forever mute, unable to do any tasks that required judgement or interpretation based on language. Of course, it was also unable to read. This meant that whenever he was faced with a page of printed matter, W.J. could read only the words on the right half of his visual field, which projected to his left hemisphere. His right hemisphere seemed blind. Reading thus became very difficult and tiring for him. He also found it impossible to write any words with his left hand, although he had been able to do so with a little effort before his operation. (He was thoroughly right-handed.)

Indeed, from the early tests on W.J. it appeared at first that his right hemisphere was nearly imbecilic. But then came the day when W.J., with a pencil in his left hand, was shown the outline of a Greek cross. Swiftly and surely, he copied it, drawing the entire figure with one continuous line. When he was asked to copy the same cross with his clever right hand, however, he could not do it. He drew a few lines in a disconnected way, as if he could see only one small part of the cross at a time, and was unable to finish the pattern. With six separate strokes, he had made only half of the cross. Urged to do more, he added a few lines but then stopped before completing it and said he was done. It was clearly not a lack of motor control, but a defect in conception – in striking contrast with the quick grasp of his non-verbal half.

Since then, a tantalizing picture of the brain's mute hemisphere has begun to emerge. Far from being stupid, the right half-brain is merely speechless and illiterate. It actually perceives, feels and thinks in ways all its own, which in some cases may prove superior. The only problem is to communicate with it non-verbally, as if it were an exceedingly intelligent animal.

There are some revealing films of the first split-brained patients to be studied in Dr Sperry's lab. (By now, eighteen patients have been tested there.) One sequence shows a twelve-year-old boy seated before a screen with his eyes fixed on a point in the centre of it. When pictures of various objects are flashed to the right or left of this point, each picture is seen only by the opposite hemisphere. A picture is flashed in the boy's left visual field, which is controlled by his right half-brain, and the boy says he saw nothing. (That, of course, is the left hemisphere speaking.) But at the same time his left hand (controlled by his right hemisphere) searches behind the screen, rejecting a wide variety of objects, until it finally finds, by touch, what it is looking for: a pair of scissors, to match the scissors that the right hemisphere saw on the screen.

In other frames, W.J. is seen trying to arrange some coloured blocks according to a diagram. He has no trouble at all doing this construction test with his left hand. But when his right hand tries, it gets hopelessly mixed up. Impatiently, his left hand shoots forward to help him, but the experimenter pushes it back. The right hand continues turning the blocks this way and that, achieving nothing. Again the left hand tries to come to the rescue, only to be pushed back. Put out, W.J. sits on that hand to keep it quiet. But he still can't do the block design with his right hand. When he is told he can try it with both hands, however, the situation grows even worse: the two hands seem to fight for control, with the right hand tearing down whatever the left hand has built.

147

In spatial abilities, the right hemisphere is clearly superior. It also recognizes faces better than the dominant left, as was shown recently with the aid of some very curious split faces developed by two of Dr Sperry's colleagues, Dr Colwyn Trevarthen, who is now at the University of Edinburgh, and Dr Jerre Levy. They cut several pictures of faces in two, then stuck some unlikely combinations together – the left side of an old man with the right side of a young woman, for instance – and flashed each composite picture briefly on a screen. The split-brained patients who were used as subjects for this experiment kept their eyes fixed on a red dot in the centre of the composite, so that the half-face in their left visual field could be projected only to their right hemisphere, and vice versa. After each composite picture had appeared on the screen, the patients were shown a choice of faces and asked to 'point to the face you saw'. Whether they used their right or left hand, they always pointed to the face matching the half that had been flashed on the left side of the screen, the half that had projected to the right side of their brain. This indicates that recognizing faces is a special ability for which the right hemisphere is dominant, the researchers believe. The left hemisphere never had a chance to select its candidate, since the right hemisphere always made the choice first. (Even in a split-brained patient, the right hemisphere can still control some movements of the right, as well as the left hand.) When, instead of pointing, the patients were asked to *tell* what they had seen, however, they made the opposite choice and described the half-face on the right, since that was the only thing their verbal side had seen. But they replied strangely, as if in a dream, explaining that they were confused. Sometimes they said, vaguely, that they didn't quite remember. However, they never once complained that there had been anything strange about the picture itself.

In general, the right hemisphere seems better at grasping the total picture, the *gestalt*, of a scene. And this talent cannot be limited to people whose brains have been split. It must be a form of specialization in all people, resulting from a division of labour much like that which gave language to the left hemi-sphere.

How many other special skills or talents are the province of the right hemisphere? Nobody knows. But many of man's more poetic or imaginative aspects may stem from there. A few years ago the Russian psychologist A. R. Luria described a composer who became speechless after a stroke, yet went on to compose better music than ever before. He could no longer *write* the notes, but he could play and remember them. Other people who lost the use of their right hemisphere remained able to speak, but could no longer remember melodies. So musical talent, too, appears to be located mostly in the right hemisphere.

Nor is the right hemisphere totally wordless, after all. With the exception of W.J., who had had more damage to his brain before his operation, the patients examined in Dr Sperry's lab have usually proved able to understand simple nouns and a few elemental verbs with their right hemisphere. Some could even add up to ten, as long as this was expressed non-verbally.

There is thus a lot of brainpower in the mute, inarticulate hemisphere. Coupled with this comes a full complement of emo-tions. One part of the film made in Dr Sperry's lab shows a young woman beginning to smile in an embarrassed way as the picture of a nude is flashed in her left visual field. When she is asked what was on the screen, however, the young woman replies that she saw nothing. Again the nude is flashed on the left side of the screen. This time the young woman blushes. A slow grin spreads across her face, and she even hides her face in embarrassment. But when asked what she saw, she again insists that there was nothing there. Pressed to explain why she was laughing, all she can say is, 'Oh, that funny machine!'

Just as the right hemisphere can make the whole face laugh (though the left hemisphere does not know why), it can make it express displeasure, even after the corpus callosum has been cut. 'This is shown in frowning, wincing, negative head-shaking and the like, in test situations where the minor hemisphere hears the major making stupid verbal mistakes – in other words, where the correct answer is known only to the minor hemisphere,' Dr Sperry has written. 'The minor hemisphere seems in such situations to be definitely annoyed by the erroneous vocal response of its better half.' At such times, though, the verbal half-brain would be unable to tell why the face to which it is attached frowned or winced, or why the head shook.

All these abilities point to the presence, in the right hemisphere, of 'a second, separate, conscious system that is definitely human in nature', as Dr Sperry put it. Nevertheless, the dominant hemisphere clearly does not trust its twin, at least in split-brained patients, and generally prefers to ignore it, if not put it down. The left hemisphere will usually deny that the left hand can do anything like retrieving, out of a bag, some object previously felt by that hand. When asked to do this for the first time Dr Sperry's subjects generally complain that they cannot 'work with that hand', that the hand is 'numb' or that they 'just can't feel anything' or 'can't do anything with it'. If the left hand then proceeds to do the job correctly, and this is pointed out to the patient, the speaking half will reply, 'Well, I was just guessing,' or, 'Well, I must have done it unconsciously.' It never even acknowledges the existence of its twin.

Much mystery surrounds the behaviour of the two half-brains in normal people. Nobody knows whether these twin halves also ignore each other, actively inhibit each other, co-operate, compete or take turns at the controls. Dr Sperry believes that they mostly co-operate, because of the 200 million fibres connecting them. But there are other opinions.

The best clues come from children and adults who have had terrible accidents. If a child's left hemisphere is destroyed by a head injury or tumour before he is five or maybe even ten years old, he can learn to speak again – sometimes after a year of silence. His right half-brain will slowly take over the job. Not so for adults, who regain some speech after a stroke only if they have enough uninjured tissue remaining near the injury, on the left side. They cannot use their right half-brain for speaking. If a young child is injured in the right hemisphere, however, he will also experience difficulty with speech, though an adult would not.

'The young child has speech and language on both sides of his head,' Dr Gazzaniga believes. 'He is, to some extent, a split brain, whose hemispheres tend to develop independently and duplicate each other.' At birth, the corpus callosum is only partly developed. It isn't until a child is about two years old that the link between his two hemispheres becomes really functional, so that everything experienced by one side is instantly available to the other. At that point, duplication of learning becomes less frequent, and true specialization begins.

By the age of ten, dominance for speech – and probably for other skills as well – is fixed. Tasks of synthesis, spatial perception and music apparently go to the right side. The left side gets all the sequential, verbal, analytical, computer-like activities. And, strangely, according to Dr Sperry, 'excellence in one tends to interfere with top-level performance in the other'. To avoid bottlenecks, eventually most of the traffic flows in one direction, while few opportunities arise for the other hemisphere to develop its own skills. The 'traffic cop' in this case may well be the corpus callosum. The speech learned by the right hemisphere in early childhood is thus functionally suppressed. In time, it may be lost or perhaps erased.

In California, recently, two young psychologists have been studying how normal people use or suppress their hemispheres. When you write a letter, for instance, does the left side of your brain show more electrical activity than the right? By pasting electrodes on the scalps of volunteers, Dr Robert Ornstein and Dr David Galin of the Langley-Porter Neuropsychiatric Institute have found that this is indeed the case, at least in right-handed people. The left side of their brains produced the characteristic fast waves of attention or activity, while the right side relaxed with slow, high-amplitude waves including the alpha rhythm. When the volunteers were asked simply to *think* about writing a letter, thus eliminating the effect of muscle movements, the pattern was exactly the same. Their right half-brain again relaxed, idle, and their left half showed fast waves. A similar pattern appeared when they read a column of print, did mental arithmetic, made up a list of verbs beginning with the letter 'R', and completed sentences. But exactly the reverse happened when they tried to reproduce designs with four-coloured blocks, remember musical tones, or draw with an Etch-a-Sketch: this time, the left side of the brain had more alpha rhythms, as if it were turned off, while the right side showed fast waves.

'Our opinion is that in most ordinary activities, we simply alternate between cognitive modes, rather than integrating them,' Dr Ornstein and Dr Galin said. 'These modes complement each other but do not readily substitute for each other.' Thus, when people are asked to describe a spiral staircase, they may begin by using words, but soon switch to hand gestures.

Ideally we should be able to turn on the appropriate hemisphere and turn off the other, whenever the task requires it. But in fact we cannot always do it. 'Most people are dominated by one mode or the other,' said Dr Ornstein. 'They either have difficulty in dealing with crafts and body movements, or difficulty with language.' Culture apparently has a lot to do with this. Children from poor black neighbourhoods generally learn to use their right hemisphere far more than the left – they outscore whites on tests of pattern recognition from incomplete figures, for instance, but tend to do badly on verbal tasks. Other children, who have learned to verbalize everything, find this approach a hindrance when it comes to copying a tennis serve or learning a dance step. Analysing these movements verbally just slows them down and interferes with direct learning through the right hemisphere.

'We don't have the flexibility we could have,' said Dr Ornstein. 'We are under the illusion of having more control than we really have.' Early in life, it seems, many of us become shaped either as 'left-hemisphere types', who function in a largely verbal world, or as 'right-hemisphere types', who rely more on non-verbal means of expression. These are two basically different approaches to the world.

So fundamental are these differences that they influence even the direction in which our eyes turn when we think. This was discovered by Dr Merle Day, of the Veterans Administration hospital in Downey, Illinois, but I heard about it from Dr Ernest Hilgard, of Stanford University, while talking to him about his work on hypnosis. Dr Hilgard suddenly stared at me, leaning close to my eyes, and said, 'Count the number of letters in Minnesota.' I did so, avoiding his gaze to concentrate better. 'You looked to the right,' announced Dr Hilgard when I finished. This meant that my left hemisphere was more easily activated than my right, he explained. Since electrical stimulation in the right side of the brain makes both eyes veer to the left, and vice versa, looking to the right while thinking showed that the left hemisphere was preferred. However, it also meant that I was not very hypnotizable, since various experiments have shown the right hemisphere to be more amenable to hypnosis. People who look to the left tend to prefer non-verbal tasks, to favour their right hemisphere and to be easily hypnotized. An unusually large proportion of those who look to the right, as I did, turn out to be scientists, researchers, writers or others who spend much of their time at analytical tasks.

Dr Ornstein and Dr Galin believe that when the habit of always using the same side of the brain becomes too pronounced, it can narrow one's personality. The two researchers are currently working on a test that may enable them to tell which half-brain a person chronically favours, and whether this habit interferes with the ability to shift dominance to the other side when necessary. They plan to try it out on people who are really specialized, such as Ralph Nader (a left-hemisphere type who has no hobbies of any kind) and right-hemisphere potters, dancers and sculptors ('preferably people who have trouble with language'). They expect to find significant differences between the two groups. This should give them a tool with which to guide

153

children or adults to new aspects of themselves, to open them to a full range of experiences.

Eventually, they hope, people will learn to activate the left or right hemisphere voluntarily. This has already been tried in their lab. With electrodes on their scalps to record changes in their brains' electrical activity, and earphones to inform them instantly of how they are doing, half a dozen volunteers have attempted to increase the asymmetry between their two half-brains. So far the results appear promising: nearly all of the volunteers have managed to activate one hemisphere more than the other, through feedback. They have produced as much difference between their two hemispheres in this way as when actually concentrating on mental arithmetic or drawing. One subject produced even more asymmetry through bio-feedback than through a change of tasks.

Some training of this kind may prove particularly useful for children who suffer from what is generally called dyslexia, or specific learning disabilities – a variety of subtle perceptual difficulties that interfere with reading, writing or spelling. About 10 per cent of the nation's children cannot process the information received from their eyes or ears with sufficient accuracy. Despite normal vision and hearing, and normal or even superior intelligence, they may confuse left and right or up and down, or give other evidence of poor co-ordination. Their symptoms have baffled doctors for years. At a conference at the National Academy of Sciences in 1969 Dr Sperry suggested that their problem may be 'an overly strong, or extensive, perhaps bilateral, development of the verbal, major-hemisphere type of organization that tends to interfere with an adequate development of spatial gnosis [knowledge] in the minor hemisphere'. If there is verbal development on both sides of the brain, the right hemisphere's special skills cannot fully emerge. At the same time, the dual verbal systems may compete for dominance in reading or writing, leading to what Dr Gazzaniga calls a problem in decision-making – 'Like a husband and wife trying to decide what to have for breakfast; one of them's got to take the lead.' If these children don't have a well-established decision system, and then receive two different interpretations of the world, they may be confused or slowed down. Through practice, they might learn to rely on one hemisphere more than the other, thus straightening out their lines of command.

All these attempts at making better use of the hemispheres' specialities pale before the urgency of aiding people who have lost one half of their brain through a stroke. The most pathetic of these patients are those who strain to speak, write, express themselves, but cannot, because the left side of their brain has been damaged by a blocked blood vessel. With only their right hemisphere available, they are speechless. Yet there is some preliminary evidence that they may be trained to communicate again, in a rudimentary way.

Surely the right hemisphere of a human being is cleverer than the whole brain of a chimpanzee, Dr Gazzaniga reasoned. And if chimpanzees can be taught to converse through sign language or plastic symbols, as they appear to have been recently (see Chapter 1), why couldn't stroke victims learn to communicate this way as well?

Fired up with enthusiasm after a visit to Santa Barbara, where Dr David Premack had taught a chimpanzee to communicate by means of plastic symbols, Dr Gazzaniga suggested to a graduate student, Andrea Velletri Glass, that she should start reading up on aphasia (the inability to speak) and prepare for a great project. For the next two years Ms Glass worked with a series of speechless patients at the Institute of Rehabilitation Medicine at New York University, half an hour a day, five days a week. Her first patient was an eighty-four-year-old woman who could neither speak nor understand speech, but who could see that Ms Glass was young and smiling at her. She responded, smiling feebly back. Ms Glass then showed her some kitchen objects: two identical pots, for instance, and a spoon. She indicated that she wanted the woman to pick out the two objects that were alike, and she repeated the procedure with two forks and a knife, and two bananas and an orange. Her patient understood very rapidly. (With chimpanzees, teaching the concepts 'same' and 'different' is a long and tedious business.) Then came the first 'word' – a green doughnut-shaped cut-out that Ms Glass had made out of construction paper. Laying out the two identical pots on a table, she placed the cut-out between them. With her mobile, expressive face, she urged her patient to do the same. It did not take the old woman long to figure out that she should insert the cut-out between all objects that were the same. She did so, with her good left hand. Her reward: a big smile and expressions of joy on Ms Glass's face. Next she learned the word 'different' – a hexagon made of orange paper. Within two months she had a vocabulary of some twelve symbols that she could pick out and place in the appropriate order to make simple statements, such as 'Andrea pours water'. She knew nouns, negatives and a question mark, but verbs were extremely difficult.

'We've had twelve patients so far,' says Dr Gazzaniga, 'and it works! That is, it works if they are still bright-eyed. If they are emotionally flat, if they don't want your smile, why should they arrange those shapes to please you?'

Dr Premack's chimpanzees have learned much more language than these patients, but only after highly intensive lessons (several hours a day) for two years, rather than short lessons for two months. This raises the possibility that the stroke victims, too, could develop a working vocabulary with which to express their basic needs and feelings. Unfortunately, Ms Glass had to stop her lessons after a short time as each patient was dismissed from the hospital and sent to a nursing home in another part of the country. The old woman, for instance, went off to Florida, and Ms Glass herself has moved to Pittsburgh. But eventually she hopes to expand this kind of programme to incorporate the whole nursing staff in a hospital, the family and, if necessary, the nursing homes where her patients will live. 'Half an hour a day is all right for experimental purposes,' she says, 'but to really help the patients, they should be encouraged to use the system twelve hours a day.' The symbols could then be made of Velcro, which sticks to a Velcro board at any angle, and the word each symbol represents could be printed on it for the benefit of all the literate people who wish to communicate with the patient.

It is not yet clear how far these patients could progress, given enough time. In part this depends on whether their memory is still good – some of them were approaching senility at the time of their strokes. But the research team was surprised to find how much most of the patients could do with their left hands: they could pick out printed words from nonsense syllables, and even spell some simple words when given cut-out letters to handle. This was far more than these global aphasics had been given credit for, and the team found it highly encouraging.

We can experience many things outside of the normal language system, as do young children before they learn to speak. Dr Gazzaniga recently tested two patients at the Cornell Medical School who were being examined for brain tumours. They were about to undergo angiograms – x-rays of their brain's blood vessels, made visible with a special dye. While a needle was in place in their left carotid artery, in the neck, to prepare them for the injection of dye, small doses of amytal (an anaesthetic) were injected into their left hemisphere, putting it briefly to sleep – a method used in many studies of brain function. The purpose was to show exactly which side their speech centre was on.

'It's a very dramatic procedure,' Dr Gazzaniga explained. 'The patient lies on a table, with both hands held in the air. Twenty seconds after the drug goes in, his right hand sinks down – he's completely paralysed on the right side, though the other side of his brain remains awake, for a minute and a half. This is our testing time. We put an object, say a cigarette, in his left hand. He feels it. His right hemisphere, which controls that hand, is wide-awake. We remove the cigarette. Then the effects of the amytal wear off and the left hemisphere wakes up. We ask the patient how he feels. "Fine," he replies. 'What did I put in your hand?' I ask. "I don't know," says the patient. 'Are you sure?'

"Yes," he says. Then we show him a series of objects – a pencil, a pad of paper, a comb, a cigarette – and ask him, "Which one was it?" In spite of everything he has said, his left hand immediately points to the cigarette.'

This shows that the memory trace, or engram, of the cigarette was encoded in his right hemisphere, and that it could be expressed non-verbally, but that the verbal side of his brain did not have access to it.

'It's a psychiatrist's dream,' Dr Gazzaniga said. 'Something that's there, in the patient's brain, and that influences his behaviour, but that he can't get at!' He believes that this may explain why memories formed in earliest childhood are inaccessible. The memories may be sharp and clear. They may control future behaviour. But since they were formed before the child learned to speak, they cannot be recalled through the language system, not even through what the Russian psychologist Lev Vygotsky called 'inner speech', speech for oneself, or thought.

Vygotsky believed that thought is born through words. Without words, he said, quoting a Russian poet, 'My thought, unembodied, returns to the realm of shadows.' Our earliest memories, too, dwell in a realm of shadows. And yet, something was experienced, and something of its flavour remains to haunt us through the rest of our lives.

Perhaps the right hemisphere's functions are too shrouded in shadows to be called thought. According to the Australian physiologist Sir John Eccles, a Nobel Prize-winner, the right hemisphere cannot truly think. He makes a clear distinction between consciousness of sounds or smells, which we share with animals, and the world of language, thought and culture, which is man-made. Animals can be conditioned, but they cannot create a culture, he claims. Primates leave no constructions, no art, nothing that can live beyond their own time, despite a brain almost as large as man's. In his opinion, everything that is truly human derives from the left hemisphere, where the speech centre is, and where interactions between brain and mind occur. When the right hemisphere of a woman whose brain has been split sees something that makes her smile or blush, it's not correct to say she can't *report* why she smiled. – she doesn't *know* why she smiled. Only the left hemisphere can have true thoughts or true knowledge, through language.

'Could the right half of the brain appreciate Chaplin's silent films?' Sir John was asked at a meeting of the Society for Neuroscience recently. 'How would you know?' he shot back, to much laughter in the audience. Both the report of such appreciation and our understanding of it would require the left hemisphere.

Nevertheless, the evidence increasingly favours a generous view of the right half-brain, whose role may be far more important than we know today.

When Einstein was asked how he arrived at some of his most original ideas, he explained that he rarely thought in words at all. 'A thought comes, and I may try to express it in words afterwards,' he said. His concepts first appeared through 'physical entities' – certain signs and more or less clear images that he could reproduce and combine. These elements were 'of visual and some of muscular type. Conventional words or other signs have to be sought for laboriously only in a secondary stage, when the mentioned associative play is sufficiently established and can be reproduced at will.' This held true only for his creative work in physics; in other activities, he had no trouble with words. He liked to compose limericks, and his letters were both fluent and pithy. Apparently he could make exceptionally good use of both sides of his brain. However, his love of music and his reliance on non-verbal concepts seem to indicate a preference for his right hemisphere.

For centuries we have concentrated largely on the verbal side of our brains: the side that produces things we know how to analyse and measure. Our mute half-brain remains uncharted. We know almost nothing about how the right hemisphere thinks, or how it might be educated – and we have just begun to discover how much it contributes to the complex, creative acts of man.

8 *Improving or destroying memory*

He is famous in neurological literature as H.M. – only his initials are given, to protect his privacy, now that everything else is gone. I dreaded meeting him, for the same reasons that I would feel guilty and embarrassed at meeting the victim of a catastrophe.

The taxi let me off before a modest row house in Hartford, Connecticut. The door opened, and there was H.M. – a tall, greying man in baggy trousers, the man for whom time stopped in 1953, during a brain operation intended to cure him of epilepsy. It was a radical operation, in which large parts of both his left and right temporal lobes (the areas around his ears and temples) were removed, and the surgeon cut unusually far into his patient's limbic system. Since then, H.M. has been unable to form new memories. It's not the past that gives him trouble – unlike some victims of amnesia, he remembers his background very clearly. It's the present he cannot grasp: everything disappears from his mind so quickly that his own life since 1953 remains a total blank.

At first glance, H.M. seemed completely normal. He greeted me at the door with a cordial smile, took my coat and ushered me to a seat in the small living room. His eighty-three-year-old mother sat down facing us. I had been told that H.M. did light assembly work in a rehabilitation centre every day, so I began by asking him whether he enjoyed his work. As H.M. hesitated, looking puzzled, his mother promptly answered for him. No, he can't go to work any more, she said, because the woman who used to drive him there moved away, 'so he just stays home'. H.M. remained silent. He began to knead his fingers nervously. I turned to him and asked whether he went out at all these days. 'He can't, because he gets lost,' his mother answered again. 'I always have to keep the door locked, or else he might walk out and never find his way back.' H.M. gestured helplessly. 'That's just it,' he said in a low voice. 'I don't remember things . . .'

He is now forty-seven years old. He cannot recognize his next-door neighbours, because his family moved to the present house twenty years ago, shortly after his operation. Once, when a psychologist who was driving him back from a medical centre asked him to help her find his house, he guided her to a street that he said was quite familiar to him, though he admitted it was not the right address. The psychologist then called his mother and learned they were on the street where H.M. had lived as a child, before his operation. During his stay at the medical centre, he had kept ringing for the night nurse, and with repeated apologies asked her again and again where he was and how he came to be there. One of the nurses fled in tears, unable to stand it any more. His doctors noted that if they walked out of the room for even a few minutes and then returned, he did not know them – they had to be introduced to him all over again.

When H.M. wants to describe his own state, he often says, 'It's like coming out of a dream, but it's getting clearer,' not realizing he has said this many times before. He ends most sentences with the phrase 'in a way'. 'I take care of the yard, in a way,' he says. Whenever he does go out to rake leaves or shovel snow, his mother must keep watching him and remind him of what he is there for.

'I just walk around, in a way,' he says. 'I don't remember other things I do habitually.' At this remark he suddenly shakes his head wonderingly and gasps, 'Boy!'

The operation that H.M. underwent had been performed experimentally once before, by the same surgeon, in an attempt to relieve a severely psychotic patient. Her memory also disappeared, but nobody noticed it – it seemed just one more symptom of her insanity. H.M., though, was clearly sane. He had above-average intelligence, a pleasant personality, a high school diploma, and for a while a good job with an electric-motor company. His only problem was his seizures. At least once a week, he suffered from grand mal attacks – terrible convulsions followed by a loss of consciousness. These had begun on his sixteenth birthday when 'he gave a w h o o, it sounded like that, and his feet straightened out, stiff as anything,' his mother recalled. 'We rushed him to the hospital – he was so stiff it was hard to get him out of the car – and he didn't come to until four hours later.' H.M. verified this. 'That's when I had my first big grand mal attack,' he said. 'That was a birthday present-and-a-half to have!' Besides these fits, he also suffered from minor attacks – momentary lapses of attention – as often as six times an hour. But the really frightening part was the grand mal seizures. 'He'd be talking to you, then he'd fall on the floor, like dead,' his mother said. Sometimes he would hit himself against the furniture as he fell.

As these attacks became more frequent, his family lived in growing fear of them. It became impossible for him to work. He took nearly toxic doses of drugs, but nothing seemed to help. Then Dr William Scoville, a neurosurgeon known for his development of a modified lobotomy called 'cortical undercutting', suggested removing part of H.M.'s temporal lobes. In desperation, his parents agreed. 'My husband talked me into it,' his mother told me unhappily, 'though I didn't like the idea.'

The operation was performed under local anaesthesia, with H.M. awake and talking throughout it all. In a sense it was a success – it did greatly reduce his epileptic attacks – but when it was over, his memory had died. Suddenly he couldn't recognize the hospital staff. Nor could he find his way to the bathroom. His real life – his ability to understand what was happening to him, to learn, to make friends – everything that mattered had come to an end.

Now H.M. sits at home, alone with his aged mother, next to old issues of the *Reader's Digest* which seem eternally new to him. Everything he reads vanishes from his mind, as if a slate had been wiped clean. He can do crossword puzzles over and over again, never remembering that he has solved them before. 'How old are you?' I asked. H.M. hesitated and looked around the room for clues. 'I think around thirty-six . . .' he replied, then somehow remembered what year it was (his mother said such memories come 'in spells') and, by subtracting his birth-date out loud, calculated that he was actually ten years older than he thought. The conversation moved on to his childhood friends. Brightening up at this reference to something he knew – the past – H.M. got up, seeking a favourite snapshot of himself with two of his friends. He went to his room and started rummaging through his drawers, desperately looking for the picture, which had been on his mirror for years. His rummaging became so frantic that finally his mother heard it from the kitchen, asked him what he wanted, and told him where the picture was. Still flustered, he brought it in. It showed him young and smiling, on a beach, a few years before his operation. One of the boys in the picture is now a physicist, his mother told me. Both have gone to college, married and led normal lives. No, she said, they never see H.M.

Dr Scoville is a busy surgeon with such a thriving practice in Hartford that sometimes he has to go without lunch. He strongly believes in neurosurgery, both of the spine (most of the cases that fill his office involve spinal nerve injuries) and of the brain. He welcomes the recent resurgence of interest in selective lobotomies and other forms of psychosurgery. He has no doubts about their morality. When he realized what his operation had done to H.M., however, he was distressed. Anxious to warn other surgeons and prevent them from treating epilepsy in the same way, he set to work publicizing the case.

First he got in touch with Dr Wilder Penfield of Montreal, the eminent neurosurgeon who had invented temporal-lobe operations for epilepsy. Dr Penfield himself had never operated on *both* sides of his patients' brains, as Dr Scoville had done, but had limited himself to one hemisphere. Nor had he had any serious problems with his patients' memory, except once, when a man inexplicably lost the ability to make new memories, much as later happened to H.M. In trying to understand this earlier case, Dr Penfield conjectured that perhaps the man had had a damaged temporal lobe on the other side (abnormal E E Gs gave some evidence of this), in which case the operation might have left him without some critical structure on either side; however, he could not prove it. So when he heard of Dr Scoville's experience 'he was very excited indeed,' Dr Scoville told me. At once he dispatched his senior experimental psychologist, Dr Brenda Milner, to Hartford to study H.M. and several other patients on whom Dr Scoville had performed similar surgery.

What Dr Milner found, and all students of neurology now know, is that the key to new memories lies in a few precious centimetres of the brain's limbic system – in the hippocampus. When surgery stopped just before the hippocampus, sparing it, the patient's memory was completely normal. If the hippocampus in one hemisphere remained intact, memory might be temporarily disrupted, but it would return. However, if both hippocampi were damaged, the loss of memory was final.

In the decades since his operation H.M. has been studied by a wide variety of psychologists, often for weeks at a time, at such research centres as M I T and the Montreal Neurological Institute. His testing has been extensive, to say the least, and the tests have turned up some interesting anomalies. Although H.M. cannot verbally recall any recent events, he still seems able to learn new motor skills. He will do a mirror-drawing or other motor task better and better, yet keep denying that he's ever seen the apparatus before. At the same time, his intellect and perceptual abilities remain intact. So does his memory for events up to about a year before his operation.

His case is uniquely 'pure-culture', the researchers say appreciatively, meaning that in the confused search for the mechanisms of memory, it appears unusually clear-cut. Yet even here there are complications: what enables H.M. to carry on an intelligent conversation, to score high on I Q tests, or to remember things for a span of nearly fifteen minutes? What allows him to recall his early life so well?

Clearly, as H.M.'s case indicates, there are several kinds or stages of memory – short-term, long-term and perhaps others in between. There must be some form of registration, then some kind of retention process and finally some system for retrieval. But what actually happens at any of these stages remains as elusive as an enigma wrapped in a mystery inside a riddle. Nevertheless, it is now possible for scientists to interrupt, or speed up, the process of memory at various stages and in many ways. At least in animals, the control of memory has become frighteningly effective, despite the primitive state of our knowledge.

A leading example of such memory research on animals is that of Dr Bernard Agranoff, a biochemist at the Mental Health Research Institute at the University of Michigan. For some time now Dr Agranoff has been inflicting a loss of memory much like H.M.'s on thousands of goldfish – all in the interest of science, to study how memory is consolidated.

New impressions are formed in only a few seconds, he explains, but unless they are fixed by some chemical process in the brain, they will fade away, much as a Polaroid picture fades unless it has been treated with fixative. 'The only way we have to study this fixation process is to disrupt it,' he said somewhat defensively. 'It's true we've tried to disrupt memory, but we really are good guys.'

He does not remove any part of the fish's brains (and, as he points out, fish don't even have a proper hippocampus). He does not destroy anything permanently. He merely injects some puromycin, an antibiotic that blocks the formation of protein, into their skulls immediately after they have learned a new skill, and the skill vanishes.

The day I visited him Dr Agranoff was expecting his weekly

165

shipment of 800 goldfish from a Missouri goldfish farm. Goldfish are quite intelligent, as fish go. It does not take them long to learn that they can avoid a mild electric shock by swimming to the other end of the tank whenever a light goes on. In Dr Agranoff's lab, in the dark, I watched a training session. Ten small fish in oblong plastic tanks were making rapid progress, as monitored by a computer: most of them crossed an underwater barrier in the middle of their tank as soon as the light flashed on, without waiting for the shock. By the end of the forty-minute session, which consisted of twenty trials, all the fish had learned it nearly perfectly. Normally, they would remember this skill for at least one month.

To obliterate this memory Dr Agranoff found that he had to inject the puromycin into their skulls immediately after the training. If he waited one hour, it was too late – the memory had been fixed. Half an hour's wait produced intermediate results, with some fish remembering to cross the barrier while others didn't.

By now, having 'used up' a couple of hundred thousand goldfish, Dr Agranoff is convinced that puromycin and similar chemicals act only on the consolidation stage of memory. 'What I think is happening is that our blocking agents block all over the brain,' he says, 'but they produce results only in those places where new protein is required to fix a new memory.' The new protein must be formed within an hour after the event, but other stages of memory are not affected. For instance, when Dr Agranoff injected puromycin into some goldfish *before* their training session, it did not interfere with the initial *learning* process – they learned to avoid shocks just as rapidly as any other fish. Three days later, however, they remembered nothing at all.

Intrigued by the implications for human beings in this method of wiping out specific memories of something just learned – of a murder, perhaps, or the location of military secrets – a reporter once asked Dr Agranoff, only half in jest, whether the CIA had been in touch with him about his work.

Dr Agranoff replied, with a smile, 'I forget.' He is quick to point out that his experiments have been limited to fish. The effects of such chemicals on man might be lethal. All he is trying to do is to learn more about the process of memory.

The idea that biochemistry is involved in the storage of memories won acceptance quite late, in the 1960s. Until then, memory was believed to be based entirely on electrical activity. Electrical circuits in the brain were supposed to lay down lasting patterns, or engrams, which produced memories. The neuropsychologist Karl Lashley spent a lifetime looking for such engrams. Convinced they must be located somewhere in the cortex, he trained thousands of animals to run mazes or learn other skills, and then systematically cut out piece after piece of their cortex, expecting that at some point this would also wipe out the memory of their training. But no matter where he cut, the memory survived – even when he removed 90 per cent of the rats' visual cortex. Finally, in 1950, after decades of struggling with the problem of how information is encoded in the brain, Dr Lashley declared in exasperation that 'the necessary conclusion is that learning just is not possible at all'.

This sense of exasperation persists, despite striking advances. The study of memory remains *the* most difficult and challenging field in the brain sciences. It has defeated, so far, the best efforts of some of the world's most imaginative scientists, including men who dropped all their previous research for its sake. It has attracted such Nobel Prize-winners as Marshall Nirenberg, Jacques Monod, Francis Crick and – perhaps most revealingly – the brilliant James Watson, author of *The Double Helix*, whose competitive instincts have been aroused by the race. The leading contenders for the key to memory are now labouring at white heat, in considerable secrecy, and fully aware of the immense possibilities involved.

If such men could crack the genetic code, why not the code of memory, which might also be cunningly embedded in some widespread, inheritable chemicals? We already know that

167

animals rely a great deal on ancestral memories, on so-called instincts that have been engraved in their brains by some genetic mechanism. A young squirrel taken away from its mother at birth and raised in isolation on concrete floors will still dig an imaginary hole in which to hide the first nut-like object it ever encounters. And even after twenty generations of breeding in laboratory cages, rats will revert to digging burrows in the ground at the first opportunity. Like these animals, the human baby is born with an impressive repertoire of abilities: it can suck, sleep, cry, salivate, kick. Its brain cells know how to organize themselves so that hunger leads to crying. The next step – learning that crying will have a certain effect, will command attention, for instance – may not be so different in kind. Robert Galambos, a physiologist of the University of California, posed this question: 'The original solution is so elegant, simple and exact; why should nature, or physiologists, abandon it in favour of some other?'

Whatever memory consists of, it must have some chemical component. Otherwise long-term memories could not survive deep freeze, hibernation, electro-convulsive shock, coma, anaesthesia or other conditions that radically disrupt the electrical activity of the brain. A chemical trace would also explain why memories are so widespread – why the engram has eluded all who have tried to find its specific location in the brain.

This is why so much excitement greeted the announcement, in 1958, that the brains of rats raised in enriched environments (where they presumably learned a great deal) were chemically different from those of rats raised in barren cages. The Berkeley team of Dr Krech, Dr Rosenzweig and Dr Bennett thus provided the first evidence of measurable biochemical changes in the brain due to experience. However, these changes could not be attributed to any single type of learning, since the rats had spent months playing with a variety of toys. Far more specific changes were reported by a Swedish researcher, Dr Holger Hydén, a few years later.

Dr Hydén found that when rats were trained to do a sort of

tight-rope act – to climb a thin wire at a steep incline to reach their food – the cells in the part of their brains that controlled balance contained 20 per cent more R N A, the nucleic acid that transmits genetic instructions. This was a striking discovery, for it opened the possibility that anything that increased the cells' R N A content might improve memory or learning, while anything that lowered the R N A level might produce forgetfulness. Dr Hydén explained that this R N A eventually gave rise to new brain protein – the very process that Dr Agranoff interrupts in his experiments with goldfish.

In memory research no 'facts' are safe, however. And as soon as a new theory is developed, it is savagely attacked by other scientists, especially by the neurophysiologists. As students of the specific connections between nerve cells in the brain, the neurophysiologists had brain research virtually to themselves until a decade ago. They remain its high priests, looking down at scientists from other disciplines who have entered their preserve. Chemists such as Dr Hydén command a certain respect from them, being considered hardheaded, though misguided (few neurophysiologists accept his findings). But their real contempt is reserved for such 'soft' scientists as psychologists, particularly those with far-out ideas. Some of them positively shudder at the name of James McConnell.

Professor McConnell, a psychologist at the University of Michigan, is the *enfant terrible* of brain research. In his spare time he edits a humourous journal, the *Worm-Runner's Digest*, which, when reversed and held upside down, becomes the scholarly *Journal of Biological Psychology*. His critics, and he has many, claim that they can't tell one from the other. The worms in the title are the tiny freshwater flatworms called planarians with which Dr McConnell won fame in the early 1960s.

He claims that worms can *eat* memories. They can learn through cannibalism, simply by eating pieces of educated relatives. 'Someday we will be able to change the educational system by synthesizing memory molecules in a test tube and

169

injecting them into kindergarten kids,' he said. 'We could probably do it right now.' He added wryly, 'I remain a controversial person. I can't imagine why . . .'

As a graduate student at the University of Texas, Dr McConnell had merely wanted to test the conventional theory that learning resulted from changes at the synapse – the junction between two nerve cells. The simplest animals to have both a brain and true synapses, planarians, were seldom used for psychological experiments, but Dr McConnell proved that they could learn to react to light when the light was followed by a mild electric shock. In the process, he was struck by his worms' extraordinary ability to regenerate: they could be cut into as many as fifty or even a hundred different pieces, and each piece would grow back into a complete worm.

What would happen if he trained a worm, cut it in half and then let each half regenerate, he wondered. Would any memory of the training be retained? A few years later, when he became a professor at the University of Michigan and had his own laboratory, he decided to find out. Two of his students, Allan Jacobson and Daniel Kimble, helped him train the tiny worms to react to light at least 92 per cent of the time. The worms were then cut in half. A month later, when all the heads had grown new tails, Dr McConnell tested them and found that they remembered as well as trained planarians which had never been cut. This was not too surprising, since their brains were unchanged. But when the tail halves, which had had to grow entirely new brains, also remembered, few people besides Dr McConnell believed the results. He concluded that specific memories were stored chemically within individual cells, not only in the brain, but throughout the animal's body.

To test his theory he tried to graft pieces of trained flatworms onto the bodies of untrained animals, but most of the animals died. Then he thought of a much simpler method: why not let the untrained worms *eat* pieces of worms that had learned to respond to the light? He knew that planarians turn cannibal when they are hungry enough. Using a particularly voracious species of planarians he proceeded to starve them for weeks, then fed them tiny, chopped-up pieces of trained animals in the hope that they would absorb memories together with the pieces.

'To our delight,' he wrote later, 'the cannibals that had eaten educated victims did significantly better (right from the very first trial) than did cannibals that had eaten untrained victims. We had achieved the first interanimal transfer of information, or, as I like to put it, we had confirmed the Mau Mau hypothesis!'

These results have now been replicated in more than twenty laboratories, in various parts of the world. But many other laboratories have failed to find any such effect, and among some conservative scientists the whole thing is treated as a joke.

'I'm ashamed of scientists, the way they're treating this issue,' said Professor David Krech, who keeps an open mind on the subject even though his own lab could not find any evidence of memory transfer. 'The accusations! There are two camps, the Believers and the Non-believers. Each side accuses the other of lying, cheating, not reporting results.'

As long as the memory-transfer experiments were limited to the lowly planarians, they could be considered a mere curiosity. It was when the arguments moved on to rats, creatures so much closer to man, that scientists were forced to take a stand. The most acrimonious dispute erupted in 1965, when Allan Jacobson reported evidence that specific memories could be injected into rats. The stakes were high. Dozens of researchers rushed to their labs to try and duplicate his results, despite the mockery of their colleagues. Within a year there appeared a seemingly polite though devastating letter in *Science* magazine, signed by twenty-three scientists from six different research labs. They had tried to repeat Dr Jacobson's experiment, they declared, but had failed in every single case. As if to illustrate the see-sawing of scientific opinion, however, one of the signers suddenly obtained positive results just as the letter was going to press. This was Dr William Byrne, a biochemist who now directs the Brain Research Institute at the University of Tennessee. Dr Byrne found that rats did learn to press a bar in a Skinner box much more easily when they were injected with RNA-containing extracts from the brains of trained animals. He published his findings shortly afterward (he remains a Believer), and so the search continued.

In 1966, Dr McConnell, who never abandoned his theories about memory transfer, began to work with rats. Rats are both more interesting and easier to train, he said. 'Besides, a lot of people wouldn't give a damn about whether you'd achieved this kind of memory transfer in worms.' He noted that only the simplest creatures, such as planarians, can literally 'swallow' learning. Men and other mammals cannot because their digestive systems would break down the food so thoroughly that the memories would be lost. Therefore, Dr McConnell trained rats to perform certain tasks, killed them, and then injected RNA-containing extracts from their brains directly into the brains of untrained rats, to see if this would make them learn the skills more rapidly. Specifically, would they learn to press the bar of a Skinner box with their chins in fewer trials? Would it take them less time to learn to jump up on a platform to avoid an electric shock? And would the extracts from the brains of rats trained for these tasks produce different kinds of behaviour? Unlike the Non-believers, he was looking for *specific* transfer of memories. A general facilitation of learning would not prove his point.

The results of these and other tests in his lab were encouraging: there seemed to be a specific transfer. But he could not shake off the controversies surrounding his work. There were always new details about the experimental procedures that might have been factors in his or other people's successes or failures – for example, how the rats had been 'gentled', or tamed, what their prior experiences had been, whether they were trained seven days a week or given a few days off. 'I won't be really happy until we have achieved a procedure that college freshmen, just reading a set of instructions, will be able to replicate successfully,' he declared. Finally he grew tired of all the arguments, and in 1972 he quit. He shut down his lab, threw out all his experimental animals, and is now devoting himself almost entirely to his other major interest – behaviour modification – in schools, hospitals and prisons. The discovery of memory transfer was premature, he believes – the field simply wasn't ready for it. 'Even if we're right, it will take a decade or so for the opinion leaders to come round.'

By now the focus of controversy about memory transfer has shifted to Dr Georges Ungar, a Hungarian-born neurochemist who believes that specific memories can be manufactured in the laboratory, with ordinary chemicals. Dr Ungar began by teaching mice to fear the dark. Normal mice always prefer dark areas to light, but those in the experimental group received electric shocks every time they entered a dark box. When he injected extracts from their brains into the abdomens of other mice, they, too, began to shun the dark almost as often as the trained animals, he reported. His next move was to find out exactly what the brain extract consisted of, chemically (he called it 'scotophobin', from the Greek *skotos*, darkness, and *phobos*, fear). Once he knew this, he asked a chemist to duplicate scotophobin, using nothing but laboratory chemicals. The synthetic scotophobin was then injected into normal rats and mice and reportedly worked nearly as well as the natural extract in making them fear the dark. At least eight laboratories are now trying to replicate this work.

Most brain scientists continue to scoff at the idea that memories can be manufactured in a test tube. 'It's a lot of baloney,' declared a neurophysiologist vehemently, 'a dead issue.' 'It's science fiction,' said a biochemist. Others reserve their judgement. 'I really don't know,' says Dr Karl Pribram, a renowned professor of neuropsychology at Stanford University. 'There may be something there – but it doesn't fit what we know.'

At the opposite extreme from the flamboyant and controversial experiments on memory transfer, and remote from the attempts to change the chemistry of memory throughout the brain, there have been some quiet but impressive advances in recent years by scientists who have focused on smaller and smaller components of the brain, in search of certainty. Theirs is a happy life, for few quarrels or accusations mar their work. On the contrary, they have won respect from nearly everyone in the brain sciences.

Their subject is often a loathsome, slimy creature from the ocean depths, a kind of sea slug called an *Aplysia*. *Aplysia* have become so popular with neuroscientists in recent years that they are in danger of becoming extinct. They owe this attention to the fact that they have relatively few but gigantic neurons – some of them almost a millimetre wide, or thousands of times larger than the neurons in the mammalian brain. This is a positive luxury, allowing researchers to insert microelectrodes into individual neurons with relative ease. It also makes it possible to pinpoint the function of each cell, to chart the cells' connections and to study the changes that occur during learning – advantages well worth the unpleasantness of working with ugly creatures that leave a trail of sticky yellow slime behind them wherever they go.

At New York University, Dr Eric Kandel, who is both a psychiatrist and a physiologist, has concentrated on five specific motor cells in the abdominal ganglion of the *Aplysia*. This ganglion, a mass of some 1,800 nerve cells, does many of the things the brain would do in a mammal: it controls the animal's heart rate and other visceral responses, as well as certain defensive reactions, such as withdrawing its delicate gill whenever nearby areas are touched. The five cells he isolated are the motor neurons that produce the gill's withdrawal. By now Dr Kandel knows them so well that he thinks of them as old friends. 'They're unique individuals!' he exclaims. 'You can give them names and spot them in every animal. They hook up together in a fairly precise way.' He has become almost as well acquainted with a family of sensory neurons and several interneurons that bring these five cells information from the outside world. Since these specific neurons are pre-wired together in every *Aplysia*, probably under genetic control, Dr Kandel has tried to find out how the neurons learn anything. It is clearly not a matter of making new connections between them in this case. What changes, then, when this group of cells learns such basic facts of life as what is important, or dangerous, and what can be safely ignored? How do they profit from experience?

The first time someone lightly touches an *Aplysia*'s skin near its fragile gill, the gill retracts and withdraws into a cavity, where it waits in safety until all danger seems past. It is a most sensible reaction. If one touches the same spot repeatedly, however, without harming the *Aplysia* in any way, the animal soon gets used to the stimulus and stops withdrawing its gill. This is a phenomenon known to psychologists as habituation. 'The same would be the case with you,' Dr Kandel told me. He suddenly slapped his palm on his desk so loud that I jumped – it sounded like a pistol shot. 'You see, you were startled! However, if I were to continue to bang, you'd think it was just a damn nuisance, and you'd ignore it,' he said. Habituation is generally considered to be the simplest form of learning. But it is highly specific, for if the stimulus changes in any way – if the *Aplysia*'s skin is touched at a slightly different spot, for instance, or with a slightly different pressure – the animal's gill withdraws just as fast as ever.

By lifting the *Aplysia*'s abdominal ganglion out through a slit in the skin, and onto a kind of illuminated stage, Dr Kandel and his colleagues have been able to study the five motor neurons at the very time these were habituating to a touch on the *Aplysia*'s skin near the gill. They found that as the animal stopped withdrawing its gill, these motor neurons stopped firing because the connections between them and the sensory neurons (which bring information from the skin) had grown ineffective. Under normal circumstances, these connections are quite effective, Dr Kandel points out. 'A learning experience can change the effectiveness of these connections from average to zero, or else to highly effective,' he explained. 'We now have examples of both such events.'

If instead of just touching the *Aplysia*'s skin lightly, one gives it a strong electric shock twice a day for ten days, the animal reacts in a manner opposite to habituation: it becomes hypersensitive. 'You can get a dramatic enhancement of the gill-reflex response,' Dr Kandel said. 'The response becomes two to eight times more powerful than in the control animal. And this makes functional sense. When an animal learns there is no danger, it is uneconomical to continue to withdraw. But with two powerful shocks a day, the animal lives in an environment that is chronically dangerous. As a result, it reacts even to a weak stimulus.'

For messages to travel in the brain as they do, flowing through millions of neurons in a split second, enough chemical neuro-transmitter must be released at the synapses to change the electrical potential of each neuron, thereby triggering off an electrical impulse that releases more neuro-transmitter at the next synapse and allows the process to start all over again. In the two decades since this system has been understood, the role of the neuro-transmitters has loomed ever larger. Now it appears, from research such as Dr Kandel's, that the amount of transmitter released by a specific neuron may vary according to previous experience. If the stimulus seems harmless, the amount of transmitter may decrease, and the animal will habituate, or stop responding. If the stimulus changes and the animal is startled again, the transmitter may flow as freely as before, and the connections between the neurons will suddenly be restored to effectiveness. If the stimulus becomes exceptionally strong and menacing, however, there will be an oversupply of chemical transmitter, and the animal will become hyper-responsive.

One key to this activity is found in the mechanism that decides what is dangerous and what is not. Such decisions require incredibly swift and complex processing, for the ganglion must remember what happened before and then compare the present stimulus with the past in order to draw its conclusions – and all this for the simplest form of learning.

Even though he is still worlds away from understanding how the ganglion does it, Dr Kandel believes that the only reliable way to learn about learning is to start with the simplest systems and work one's way up. One can start at an even more elementary level: Marshall Nirenberg and others are now studying how a single cell accumulates neuro-transmitters, for instance. Instead of isolating a few cells in a live animal, they work in tissue culture, measuring the minute changes in a single cell as it reacts to transmitters from another cell – in a dish.

Eventually Dr Kandel hopes to use sea slugs and other simple animals to develop models that might shed light on mental illness. If animals can learn to be hyper-responsive, it should be possible to produce chronically anxious, neurotic *Aplysia* or squid. Several different mental diseases could be modelled in this way. Since the animals' nervous systems would be known intimately, the changes that occur in them as they become disturbed and also during recovery could be observed in great detail. Various therapies might be tried on them. Considering how much of mental illness remains a mystery, such models might be a major contribution to research.

Whether they choose to study the memory of a few cells, as does Dr Kandel, of fish, as does Dr Agranoff, or of human beings, as in the case of H.M., the scientists who try to decipher memory seldom tackle the biggest problem of all: how the brain *codes* events so that they can be stored, compared and recalled. Some such code must underlie all processing in the brain. Yet most researchers simply assume that it exists and work around it, looking for evidence of memory in the animal's behaviour or in his brain's chemicals. The code itself seems beyond our comprehension, and thinking about it can drive one crazy, according to the few psychologists, such as Professor George Miller of Rockefeller University, who have tried to establish a beachhead in this field. Not only do we fail to understand the brain's extraordinary filing system, but we have no explanation for Lashley's finding that memories survive nearly all brain injuries. The memory file is at once accurate and subtle and widely distributed throughout the brain.

Recently, Karl Pribram suggested a new approach, based on what he calls 'the most sophisticated principle of information storage yet known: the principle of the hologram'. This was originally developed by the physicist Dennis Gabor in the 1940s to improve the quality of photographs taken through an electron microscope. The hologram requires laser light, which shines in a pure, straight beam rather than spreading in all directions as does ordinary light. The laser light from a single source must be split into two parts, so that one part is bounced back by an object or scene, while the other part interacts with this reflection. The resulting interference pattern is recorded on film. This is the hologram. It does not look like the original subject at all, but it has a great virtue: 'If even a small corner of a hologram is illuminated by the appropriate input, the entire original scene reappears,' explains Dr Pribram. 'Moreover, holograms can be layered one on top of the other and yet be separately reconstructed.' If memories are stored in similar 'neural holograms' caused by the interaction of different nerve impulses, Dr Lashley's findings suddenly make sense.

Dr Pribram thinks that we remember scenes from our past in a two-stage process. Some stimulus – a glimpse, a sound or perhaps a taste – triggers a short-term memory mechanism, which searches through our enormous file of holograms for the best fit. When it finds some association, 'large segments of the holographic mechanism become involved, the zoom is extended so that attention is focused on one or another detail; attention is concentrated'. He points out that several images can be superimposed on a single holographic plate, on successive exposures, so efficiently that some ten thousand million bits of information can be stored usefully in a cubic centimeter. Yet each image can be retrieved immediately and with ease, without being affected by any other. No other coding mechanism known to man can equal this performance and, so far, none can come closer to matching the brain's ability.

It is an attractive hypothesis, perhaps even correct. Several new bits of evidence about the sensitivity of brain cells fit in with it. But we may not known the truth for generations.

Regardless of how it is encoded, however, everything we do leaves a trace in our brains. Every event, every emotion or experience is permanently engraved, even if we never summon it to awareness. It must be there somewhere, awaiting only the right stimulus to appear, as the monumental work of Wilder Penfield has shown.

In 1936 a sixteen-year-old girl sat, wide-awake, on an operating table at the Montreal Neurological Institute. Her skull had been opened under local anaesthesia, and now Dr Penfield and his associates were trying to locate the area in her right temporal lobe that set off her major epileptic attacks. They stimulated here and there, painlessly, with their electrodes. Suddenly the girl cried out, 'Someone coming towards me!' It seemed so real that she thought it was actually happening. When Dr Penfield stimulated another point in her brain, she said she heard the voices of her mother and her brothers.

Nothing of the kind had ever been seen before. Dr Penfield, who had carefully mapped the cortex of hundreds of patients, knew that stimulation in the auditory area could produce ringing or buzzing sounds – but never voices that speak. Stimulation in the visual area might make patients see stars of light or moving colours – but not 'someone coming towards me'. Until then, only the *elements* of sensation had been called forth by man's electrodes. But here was a complete hallucination, or dream, which reproduced specific experiences from the girl's early childhood. It was, in fact, the same dream that always preceded her epileptic attacks.

In the following decades, the tireless Dr Penfield studied the living brains of more than a thousand patients. In forty cases, all of them epileptics, he found the same sudden 're-experiencing'

179

of the past when an electrode gently stimulated a part of the temporal lobe that he called the 'interpretive cortex'.

'Oh, gosh! There they are, my brother is there,' exclaimed a twelve-year-old boy during such stimulation. 'He is aiming an air rifle at me . . .' When stimulated a little later, he said, 'My mother is telling my brother he has got his coat on backwards. I can just hear them.' Afterwards, he explained that these were real memories, of things that had actually happened, but that during the brain stimulation they had seemed 'more real' than memory.

With an electrode touching her interpretive cortex, a young woman heard an orchestra playing a popular tune so clearly that she thought the radio had been turned on. She hummed along with the tune, at what seemed a normal tempo, whenever she was being stimulated; everyone in the operating room recognized the song. But she stopped as soon as the electrode was removed. 'Over and over again, restimulation at the same spot produced the same song,' reported Dr Penfield, and 'all efforts to mislead her failed'.

A young man suddenly felt 'as though I was in the bathroom at school', years before. A secretary experienced being in an office. 'I could see the desks,' she reported minutes after the stimulation stopped. 'I was there, and someone was calling to me, a man leaning back on a desk with a pencil in his hand.' Stimulation at a nearby spot made her see 'the place were I hang my coat up when I go to work'.

The experiences called up by electrodes placed at nearby points were always similar, but those brought on by stimulation at widely separated points in the interpretive cortex had little in common. One patient, who had arrived from South Africa only a month before, exclaimed, in great surprise, 'Yes, doctor, yes, doctor. Now I hear people laughing – my friends in South Africa!' Asked about this, he explained that he seemed to be laughing with his cousins, Bessie and Ann, whom he had left behind on a South African farm, though he knew he was now on an operating table in Montreal. When he was stimulated at a point fully two centimetres away, however, the scene changed abruptly – he heard a Canadian song.

There is in every human mind a mechanism that records the stream of consciousness, Dr Penfield concluded. Normally, when a man tries to retrieve something from his past, he remembers only generalizations – 'If this were not so, he might be hopelessly lost in detail.' But no matter how unimportant, the experiences described by his patients were as sharp and detailed as if 'a strip of cinematographic film with sound track had been set in motion within the brain'. They were the kind of experiences that normally slip rapidly beyond the range of voluntary recall. In his patients they could be summoned either during an epileptic fit or during electrical stimulation of the brain. Dr Penfield explained that once a local epileptic irritation has lowered the threshold for a specific pattern of electrical activity, any excitation of the grey matter in that area will set off the same response. This is why his electrodes called forth memories only in people who had epilepsy. The epilepsy made their brains easier to stimulate, though it did not in itself produce the stream of consciousness.

'It is clear enough that we are activating a normal mechanism in the brain,' Dr Penfield declared. This mechanism can bring forth a vivid recollection of the past, though where it is and how it works remain unknown. He noted that sometimes one runs into a person one hasn't seen for many years and is struck by a sudden sense of familiarity, even before one has time to 'think'. 'The opening of this forgotten file was subconscious,' said Dr Penfield. 'It was not a voluntary act. You would have known him even against your will. Although Jones was a forgotten man a moment before, now you can summon the record in such detail that you remark at once the slowness of his gait or a new line about the mouth.' It was all there.

Such feats of memory indicate a highly efficient filing system in the brain, which allows related experiences to be classed together and then cross-indexed. One of Dr Penfield's patients seemed to have a mental file for the concept of 'grabbing' or

'snatching', for instance. Any event suggesting a boyhood experience in which something was yanked away from him would
trigger off a major epileptic attack. The actual memory of this
incident brought on a fit; but so did seeing a child take a stick
from the mouth of a dog, or an officer grab a rifle from a cadet
on parade, or a man snatch his hat from a hat-check girl. Apparently, the same kind of filing system was used both to evaluate the present and to tap into the stream of consciousness. In
certain epileptics, the shock of recognition might produce an
attack. In normal people, a matching stimulus can sometimes
open up a long-forgotten file, laying out its contents in all their
fullness, as happened to Proust when he felt the sweet taste of
a *madeleine* in his mouth and remembered every detail of his
visits to an aunt in his youth. Similarly, under hypnosis, people
can suddenly remember many events or even speak foreign
languages they thought they had utterly forgotten. In some cases,
they can recall what they heard while apparently unconscious,
under anaesthesia, during an operation. (One woman never for-
gave her surgeon for what he said during her hysterectomy:
'Well, that takes care of this old bag' – even though he was
referring to the organ he had removed, and not, as she thought,
to her.)

Despite its wealth of details, this kind of memory may have
definite limits, as Dr Penfield discovered to his surprise after
analysing all his cases afresh in 1963. Some things were absent:
during the brain stimulation, his patients never remembered
speaking, for instance – only listening. They never relived the
experiences of writing a letter, adding up figures, making a
decision, eating, drinking or making love. They never *acted* –
they only watched others act. Most of the time, it seemed, they
heard music or voices, or saw people from their past. Baffled,
but not discouraged, Dr Penfield concluded that the missing experiences might well be recorded elsewhere in his patient's
brains. By stimulating their temporal lobes, he was tapping into
the stream of consciousness at only one place; other techniques
might reach deeper parts of the stream. And even though he had

no certain evidence that the record was complete, at least he had shown that it existed.

The stream of consciousness may be filled with trivia that cannot be recalled voluntarily, but once a recollection has emerged from this stream and won a place as an established memory, it is nearly invulnerable. Dr Lashley's work and countless more recent experiments are good evidence of that. Then how do people forget? This, too, remains shrouded in mystery. However, psychologists have noted that the process of forgetting is generally linked to some sort of interference – to a strong stimulus that disrupts the old memory, either by weakening it or by substituting another memory in its place. If so, it might be possible to dislodge unwanted, painful memories deliberately. Dr Murray Jarvik, professor of pharmacology and psychiatry at UCLA, believes that one could dredge up the old memory – the phobia, or the nightmare – and interfere with it at the very moment of its emergence into consciousness, either through a vivid impression of something similar but benign, which would eventually replace it, or through amnesic drugs. There must be a chemical step involved whenever a memory is retrieved, Dr Jarvik points out; therefore, drugs should be able to affect it. Selective amnesia might then become a valuable tool of psychotherapy. But Dr Jarvik warns that such things are still far off in the future.

A much more likely development in the near future is the introduction of drugs that can improve man's memory.

We already know how to make animals learn more quickly, by sharpening their memory with chemicals. A dozen different substances will do the job. They are all dangerous stimulants, such as strychnine (a poison), metrazol (a convulsant) and amphetamine (the addictive 'speed' that kills), but animals can tolerate them in small doses. Similar but safer drugs may soon become available for human use.

When a drug such as strychnine is given *before* an animal's training session, the animal performs better. Karl Lashley proved this half a century ago. However, Dr Lashley's experiments were difficult to interpret. The drug might simply make the animals more alert, or more eager for the food reward; it did not necessarily improve their ability to learn. In the late 1950s a young psychobiologist, Dr James McGaugh, found his curiosity aroused by reports that electro-convulsive shocks could make rats forget what they had just learned. Presumably, the shocks disrupted the consolidation of memory (as did Dr Agranoff's injections of puromycin in fish). If so, he reasoned, could stimulants such as strychnine have the opposite effect? Would they *improve* the consolidation of memory during its soft, unjelled stage? To find out, he decided to inject the drugs *after* the training session rather than before. He was immediately successful. His mice learned to run a maze far better when they received an injection of strychnine as much as one hour after their training session. The more strychnine he gave them, up to a point, the better they learned. Instead of going to the wrong arm of a maze about twenty-five times before grasping that they had to choose the white alley at every turn, the mice that had received the largest dose of the drug learned after only five or six errors. From the scientist's point of view, the nicest thing about the experiment was that the animals had no strychnine in their systems either at the time of training or at the time of retest. Thus the drug could not have affected their alertness or motivation. It acted directly on their memory.

Equally dramatic results were obtained with metrazol and with amphetamine, although these had to be injected within fifteen minutes of the training. After trying several different drugs, in graduated doses, at varying times and with different kinds of learning tasks, Dr McGaugh concluded that he had made his case. 'The robust nature of the effect is beyond question,' he declared. 'The effects are as long-lasting as those of ordinary memory. What we produce is either a quicker or a stronger consolidation of memory, so that whatever is learned, it's learned better.'

The drugs could even bring back memories that appeared to

have been erased by electro-convulsive shock. 'We can now block and unblock,' said Dr McGaugh, who is Chairman of the Department of Psychobiology at the University of California at Irvine. 'If we produce retrograde amnesia by electro-shock, we can undo it with drugs. But all this is time-dependent. We must administer the excitant within a short period of time after the inhibitor.'

This made him doubly curious about what the electro-shock actually did to his animals' brains. It turned out that a current strong enough to produce amnesia (and seizures) also prevented new protein from being formed in the brain – the same process that Dr Agranoff has interrupted in fish.

'The brain cells are supposed to be storing information,' said Dr McGaugh. 'But in the meantime we distract them with a lot of electrical current, and at some point they say, "I can't attend to what I'm supposed to be storing if you yell at me all the time." Essentially I think that's what's happening – so the animal has seizures, and a 30 per cent reduction in brain protein synthesis, and also amnesia.'

At that point someone noticed a peculiar after-effect: for several hours after the seizures, the mice had abnormal brain waves. Their E E Gs showed almost none of the slow theta waves that normally occur intermittently in the brain. Intrigued by the lack of this mysterious brain rhythm, which is so often connected with learning, a graduate student in Dr McGaugh's lab decided to forget about the seizures and just look for theta waves. He discovered that the more theta waves appeared in an animal's E E G after a training session, the more it remembered. This was true in all cases – when the electric shocks to its brain were strong enough to provoke seizures as well as when they were too weak, and also when no shock was administered at all. Apparently, the best predictor of memory was the amount of theta waves recorded in the animal's brain.

Dr McGaugh now tells his students that 'if you want to learn, and you're a rat, it's a good idea to have some theta'. But he does not believe the theta waves are a sign of memory as such.

185

Rather, they show that the brain is in the right state to process and store information. To bring back another missing link, the theta waves seem to come mostly from the hippocampus, the critical structure that was removed from H.M.'s brain. It may be that in order to learn and remember, one needs to have theta in the hippocampus.

As soon as the results of Dr McGaugh's first experiments became known, people began to talk about 'get smart' pills and learning drugs. The fact that he produced greater gains with 'stupid' rats from a maze-dull strain than with 'clever' rats from a maze-bright strain led some desperate parents to hope that he had found a cure, at last, for their mentally retarded children, and that pills could give them normal IQs. 'I had to spend months writing to distraught parents that there was nothing I could do for their children,' Dr McGaugh said despondently. Drugs cannot change higher-level conceptual abilities, he pointed out – they can only improve memory. And being able to memorize the multiplication table does not mean that you can solve problems using it. He now plays down the implications of his research for mental retardation, so as not to arouse any false hopes.

On the other hand, there is a group that may someday benefit enormously from his work: the aged. Many otherwise healthy old people suffer from a frightening loss of memory. There is an element of H.M. in all of them. 'My mind is like a sieve,' complains an old woman I know. 'I don't remember anything I read in the newspaper – don't know why I read it. But I remember clearly what happened long ago . . .' When this loss becomes extreme, it foreshadows the total deterioration seen in thousands of miserable, confused, incontinent and withdrawn senile patients in the back wards of mental hospitals. Yet there is good evidence that such loss of memory might be prevented, or even reversed, with drugs. Several experiments with ageing mice and rats have shown that they are far more responsive to memory drugs than younger animals. With young rats, for instance, amphetamine must be injected within fifteen minutes after a training session to have any effect. With ageing rats, there is an improvement in memory even when the drug is injected two hours later. Evidently, they take that much longer to consolidate their memories. The process might then be speeded up and sharpened with drugs.

'I put my money on the aged,' said Dr McGaugh. 'At least you know what memory they had, what memory they've lost, and when they've lost it. So you can try to reinstate it – that's quite different from putting in something that was never there.'

Not surprisingly, several pharmaceutical companies are now racing to develop a good memory drug. Field tests of various kinds have been going on for several years, in deepest secrecy. The most sensational of these experimental drugs, the inosines, sound too good to be true: not only would they make people remember and learn better, but they would also kill viruses and treat illnesses for which there is no present cure. The researchers involved refuse to describe them further.

Meanwhile, the most enthusiastic believers in bio-feedback have found a new goal: training people to produce more theta waves voluntarily, so as to improve their memory. Of course, they have yet to distinguish clearly between the kind of theta activity that is involved in memory and the kind that has been linked to such disparate conditions as reverie and annoyance. Then they must learn to control it. But they are not discouraged.

Will it then become possible to turn memory on or off, at will? There is good reason to believe so. We will be able to use either drugs or bio-feedback. We will know how to enhance certain experiences, making them more vivid and easier to play back, while deliberately obliterating the memory of others. Even today, when doctors must perform some painful medical procedures during which they cannot put their patients to sleep, they use amnesic drugs such as Valium. Valium is a common tranquillizer when taken by mouth, but when injected into the veins, it makes people forget. 'They're not unconscious,' Dr Jarvik explained. 'They do suffer – real pain! But afterwards, they don't complain about it.' In the future, we may decide to resemble H.M. temporarily, before events so horrible that we do not wish any permanent record of them.

What we seek in life is usually the opposite: a heightening of experience. This we could get by sharpening our memory for special occasions. The brain scientists are rapidly approaching the time when they can provide it for us – if not in youth, at least before we lose our memory in old age.

9 The control of violence

In these violent times, when murders and muggings are so common as to pass almost unnoticed, there is a deep longing for some simple, physical solution to overwhelming social problems. This is one reason why the brain scientists' work on violence holds such fascination. Can they invent a pill that would control all violence? Or devise brain operations to prevent people from going berserk?

Even a president of the American Psychological Association, Dr Kenneth Clark, recently suggested that some form of medication, which he called 'internal disarmament', should be given to world leaders to preserve peace. Noting the great advances in the brain sciences, he placed his hopes in the products of research. But many scientists question the need for such tampering with the brain. Dr Karl Pribram exclaimed after hearing Dr Clark's speech, 'The normal brain is beautiful! There is no demoniacal animal or force lying within that needs chemical treatment.'

Some cultures are violent; others are not. A child's earliest environment plays a major role in setting his level of violence. After that, education, ideology, example and circumstances do the rest – assuming that the brain is normal.

In the brain, violence is turned on by mechanisms that scientists are only beginning to understand. Since gaining access to the deeper parts of the brain which control emotions, particularly the hypothalamus and the limbic system, they have discovered some of the more important triggers. They have produced rage in otherwise peaceful cats and rats, just by injecting some chemicals into various parts of their hypothalami. They have provoked attacks by electrical stimulation of monkeys' brains. And they have come to realize that violence can sometimes result from physical, as well as psychological, causes.

The extra y chromosome found in about two out of every 1,000 men has been blamed for a variety of crimes, though the effects of this characteristic on the brain are still far from clear. In addition, thousands of people suffer from various kinds of brain damage that may predispose them to sudden acts of violence. The limbic system is the most vulnerable part of the brain, declared Dr Frank Ervin, now a professor of psychiatry at U C L A. Poor prenatal or obstetrical care, car accidents, falls and other injuries can leave permanent scars in it. So can various chemicals. When this area is damaged, people may over-react to stress.

'They are the ones who cause traffic accidents and deaths on the highway,' Dr Ervin pointed out. 'They may get along all right for long periods of time, but in situations that would make you irritated, and me angry, they lose control.' This has nothing to do with the healthy aggression of an 'aggressive salesman', he explained. He was not talking about angry feelings or words, nor even actions that can harm someone indirectly, but about direct, face-to-face physical attacks on other people, with the intent to injure – the kind of violence that stands out because it is far above the accepted cultural level.

In the United States, this cultural norm is set much higher than in some other countries. On a visit to Japan, Dr Erwin was surprised to learn how little it takes to brand one as violence-prone in a nation where many people commit suicide, but few attack one another. (In warfare against foreigners, of course, they obey different laws.) When he asked some Japanese colleagues whether they had any patients violent enough to warrant brain surgery, they said yes, and showed him around the hospital wards. The first patient he saw was a man who had been brought to the doctors' attention simply because he had been in a fight in a bar on a Saturday night. 'My hair stood on end,' Dr Ervin recalled. He was aghast that such behaviour could be considered a symptom of extreme violence. Yet when he asked the doctors for more information on the case and looked over the man's brain-wave tracings, x-rays and other records, he discovered that this was exactly the same kind of brain-injured person he'd been treating in Boston. The same brain abnormalities that made a Japanese get into a brawl apparently led Americans to launch murderous attacks. 'Doing cross-cultural neurosurgery would be very confusing!' said Dr Ervin. 'What I'm concerned with, and they were too, is the guy who exceeds the norm.'

In Dr Ervin's definition, armed robbery does not qualify as exceptional violence – at least not in the United States. 'Among people who earn their living robbing banks, killing is very rare,' he said. Occasionally they may kill out of panic, to make an escape, but in general they commit no more murders than do bank tellers. The average city mugger does not *seek* violence, either. He is usually a drug addict who needs money to support his habit, and his actions are quite cold-blooded, in a predatory way.

Nor is Dr Ervin concerned with the deliberate violence of revolutions and warfare – the kind that makes people kill innocent bystanders, or throw napalm on women and babies, for ideological reasons. 'Under normal circumstances, in face-to-face confrontation with another human being, *perceived* as a human being, there are biological constraints built in against killing him. There is no culture where it's not a part of the ethos that you don't kill an opponent when he's down.' At My Lai, the soldiers had stopped perceiving the villagers as human beings because of the panic, confusion and ambiguity of the total environment, he believes. He doubts that Lieutenant William Calley, who was convicted of murdering Vietnamese civilians in 1968, had any appreciable brain damage. 'On the other hand, some of *my* boys became heroes in the war!' he said. 'They won Distinguished Service Medals – for blowing their top.'

191

Even if all these somewhat loose categories are eliminated, there is still a large group of otherwise normal people who suffer from what Dr Ervin calls 'episodic dyscontrol' because of subtle and localized damage to their brains, and who can become extremely violent without provocation.

Their kind of violence is a medical problem and should be treated as such – with drugs or, in extreme cases, brain surgery, Dr Ervin believes. However, it is seldom recognized by doctors, and treatment is largely unavailable. 'Right now, if a fellow is unusually violent, people call a cop, a lawyer, a minister, a social worker – anyone but a doctor,' he says. In his opinion, many of the senseless crimes that fill the pages of our newspapers could be eliminated by giving such people medical treatment.

Among the few specialists who advocate direct action on the brain to control fits of violence, the team of Dr William Sweet, chief of neurosurgery at Massachusetts General Hospital, Dr Vernon Mark, director of neurosurgery at Boston City Hospital and, until recently, Dr Ervin, who directed the Stanley Cobb Laboratories of Psychiatric Research at Massachusetts General Hospital before moving to California, has taken a leading role.

Despite its impressive credentials – all these men also teach, or have taught, at Harvard Medical School – the team has become rather controversial, both because of the operations it has performed on violent epileptics and because of fear that the techniques it pioneered might be applied to other kinds of violent persons as well. Even the team members' own colleagues have sometimes joined in the criticism. The crux of the question has been whether their operations are really surgery for the relief of intractable epilepsy, or whether they represent a new form of more precise psychosurgery, designed to control unpleasant behaviour.

The team firmly maintains that its patients' attacks of violence are directly related to temporal-lobe epilepsy – are, in fact, symptoms of it. The doctors also want it made quite clear that they don't run a production line. 'You won't see a lot of people walking around with wires in their heads,' Dr Ervin pointed out when I called to make an appointment. 'We have none at the moment, and never more than one or two at any time. Lots of people come in for diagnosis and drugs; that, yes. But operations? We're very chary about that.'

In the past seven years the team has operated on a total of thirteen epileptic patients to reduce their violence. In all cases they began by using anti-convulsant drugs and other therapies, moving on to surgery only when their other efforts had failed. Even then, the team's first step was always to take extensive recordings, for several weeks, from electrodes inserted into the patient's brains. Only after this was done did they begin the actual treatment: the destruction of specific cells in the patients' amygdala, a part of the limbic system.

There was, for instance, a rather pale but otherwise ordinary-looking young man who walked into Boston City Hospital a couple of years ago. Quiet and polite, he gave straightforward answers to the doctor's questions about his age (twenty) and his seizures, which had begun when a gang of boys knocked him out on his way home from school. After his routine interview, he was taken to a ward on another floor – and suddenly flew into a rage. Grabbing a strap with a heavy buckle, he struck one nurse savagely, flailed at others, tore at the barred windows, and managed to fight off four male attendants until the police subdued him with a chemical spray.

Six weeks later, he was in the operating room, sitting up but actually asleep, his chin resting on his chest. Only the glistening top of his head protruded from the green sheets and the towels that enveloped him. Dr Mark leaned over his bare, shiny skull and pierced a hole in it with a surgical drill. Through this hole he injected some radiopaque dye to allow more accurate x-rays of the boy's brain. Then he placed a rigid, curved frame a few inches over the skull, nailing it into position with three metal pins that he tapped into the scalp.

'This stereotactic machine will guide our fine-wire electrodes to their target deep in the brain,' Dr Mark explained in a film of the operation. 'This is our target right here [he pointed to a

G

spot in the x-ray picture, representing the boy's amygdala – a tiny, almond-shaped structure deep behind the temple]. We'll use our plotting chart to translate the measurements from the x-ray to a "phantom", an exact duplicate of the machine, and lock the electrode on target before transferring it to the real machine on the patient's head."

A close-up of the hole in the boy's skull showed some blood oozing out of it, then the electrode entered the brain. 'When the collar of the lever arm lies down flat, we're ten millimetres away from the target,' Dr Mark explained as he showed me the film. 'Now we're recording from the tip of the electrode in the brain. See some abnormal brain waves there? [He pointed to a row of jagged tracings on a graph.] We're adjusting the position . . . The electrode is now in the proper position in the left amygdala. It can stay in safely for weeks or months. We'll put some dental cement around it to keep it in place – it's sterile and fills up the hole. Then we'll stimulate his brain with a weak electric current through ten different points along the tip of the electrode, until we find the exact spot where stimulation will reproduce the abnormality.'

Having identified a clump of cells in this way, Dr Mark burned them out with a small burst of electricity.

Before his operation, the boy had had attacks of 'bad temper' at least twice a week. He would smash furniture or beat people. 'When I'm in an argument or something like that, it gets me mad,' he told the doctor. 'Once I woke up like in a dream. I got up, and felt my feet were bigger. I thought I was a monster, they were so big. So I took a table and flung it right up the wall.' He also had convulsions, during which he would lose consciousness. According to Dr Mark, the surgery stopped his major epileptic seizures (though it did not eliminate minor spells), and it prevented his attacks of rage – at least for a while. In fact, for several months he didn't seem able to defend himself very well against people he had previously terrorized. He let his younger brother beat him up. He went to work in a shoe factory, the first job he had ever held, and did quite well for nine months. Then 'those feelings' began to come back – the same ones that used to announce his epileptic seizures. One day, when a fellow worker kidded him about his 'puny' size, he suddenly lost control again, lunged at him and broke the man's jaw. So now he is a candidate for another operation, to destroy the amygdala on the other side of his brain.

The amygdala is most suspect in such cases because it seems most directly related to violence, though several other parts of the brain, including the hypothalamus, are also involved. The wildest lynx or bobcat will become tame after its amygdala has been removed, and killer rats will no longer attack mice. Any lingering doubts about the amygdala's role in violence were removed by an ingenious experiment in which a monkey's brain was operated on so that its right eye sent information only to the right hemisphere, and the left eye sent messages only to the left hemisphere. Its corpus callosum, which connected the left and right hemispheres, was also cut, and only the right amygdala was removed. This created a truly schizoid monkey – unusually docile and tame when approached from the right, but as cowering or aggressive as before the operation when approached from the left.

After this experiment, it was inevitable that someone would try similar surgery on human beings. Instead of removing the entire amygdala, however, selected parts of it could be burned out through fine-wire electrodes. Brain surgery to correct violence began in the early 1960s, in Japan, in an institution for the mentally retarded. Dr. H. Narabayashi went at it in a big way – he operated on ninety-eight mentally retarded and assaultive persons of various ages – but the results were not brilliant. Of thirteen adults in the series, only four were clearly improved, three improved temporarily but relapsed within a few months or a year, and six were not improved at all. However, a precedent had been set.

In the United States, Professor R. R. Heimberger, of the University of Indiana, was the first to follow Dr Narabayashi's example, operating on twenty-five severely epileptic and violent patients. He claims to have eliminated violence in seven cases and reduced it in sixteen others, leaving only two unimproved. Since then, surgeons in Denmark, France, India and Mexico have done similar operations, as has the Boston team. Japanese surgeons who work with assaultive brain-injured children have begun to bypass the amygdala and destroy instead a small portion of the hypothalamus – a technique they call 'sedative surgery'.

Although there is considerable evidence that abnormal violence can be reduced by destroying some parts of the limbic system, at least in certain cases, it does not always work, either because the abnormality may be much more widespread, or because it may have entirely different origins. The limbic system is still very poorly understood. Even the amygdala, one of the largest, most accessible and best-studied structures in the limbic system, remains in many respects a mystery.

'We need to know our goal more precisely,' said Dr Ervin. 'What is the least intervention that will modify behaviour in certain ways? If it is to kill ninety-four cells in that corner, it could be done with a proton beam, *without surgery*. You set the beam so that the protons give up all their energy at a certain distance, at the so-called Bragg peak, without damage to any tissue before that point. It's a lovely, lovely method! It's the technique of choice for removing a cancerous pituitary nowadays, because it does not require surgery. If we knew for sure what to destroy, we could do it that way.'

Meanwhile, surgeons who believe in the value of such operations must rely on the clumsier technique of placing electrodes inside the brain to locate the points they are looking for. This is done by stimulating various spots with a weak electric current and studying the behaviour that results.

An extraordinary film of this procedure shows Dr Mark probing the brain of a young woman, selecting various points by remote control, while she is wide-awake. The daughter of a professor, she had spent most of her life in prisons, mental hospitals and institutions for the criminally insane. She had tried to commit suicide four times. She had nearly killed two women – one of them a girl who accidentally brushed against her in the ladies' room of a cinema, and whom she stabbed in the heart. She had attacked at least ten other people without apparent provocation. All this violence apparently resulted from brain damage, which could be traced to a severe case of encephalitis following an attack of the mumps when she was eighteen months old. Yet none of the existing anti-seizure drugs or tranquillizers could reduce her spells of rage. She had defeated the best efforts of three of the nation's leading medical centres, receiving years of therapy, and even shock treatments, to no avail. Finally she had been taken to Massachusetts General Hospital to see Dr Mark, who implanted two sets of electrodes in her brain and connected them to a stimoceiver placed on top of her head so she would be free of trailing wires. Dr José Delgado had made this device available to the Boston team. Without a stimoceiver, the electrodes in her brain would have had to be connected to electrical equipment in the laboratory. Now, no longer restricted by the fear of tearing out some wires and injuring her brain, the patient could move about freely. At the same time, the doctors could receive messages of her brain's electrical activity, or stimulate various points in her brain, from a distance of up to one hundred feet – without her knowledge, since brain tissue itself is incapable of sensation.

As the film opens, the patient, a rather attractive young woman, is seen playing the guitar and singing 'Puff, the Magic Dragon'. A psychiatrist sits a few feet away. She seems undisturbed by the bandages that cover her head like a tight hood, from her forehead to the back of her neck. Then a mild electric current is sent from another room, stimulating one of the electrodes in her right amygdala. Immediately, she stops singing. The brain-wave tracings from her amygdala begin to show spikes, a sign of seizure activity. She stares blankly ahead. Suddenly she grabs her guitar and smashes it against the wall, narrowly missing the psychiatrist's head.

In another sequence, she is shown smiling and chatting

197

amiably with her psychiatrist when, without warning, she begins to scowl. She bares her teeth, then suddenly, so rapidly that the eye can barely follow her, she springs at the wall and hammers it with her fists and head. Watching the film, I was taken by surprise even though I knew what to expect. It was like a snake striking – so swift that I gasped.

Dr Ervin pointed out that although these attacks looked wild and uncontrolled, the patient never hurt the psychiatrist. 'Having lost contact, she turned and beat against the wall, instead of the human whom she knew and towards whom she had ambivalent feelings,' he said. Brain stimulation can turn on anger or rage, but it cannot dictate how these emotions will be expressed.

In twenty years of working with the most violent patients in hospitals and prisons, Dr Ervin has never been attacked. The fact that he is six feet four inches tall may help, but he credits his non-aggressive manner. 'I always sit down, never stand up while talking to a violent patient,' he said. 'One should never be alone with such a patient in a small room; there should be lots of people, much space, and a calm atmosphere.

'I don't find them a threatening group,' he continued. 'They're scared people! A lot of what we identify as aggressive is in fact defensive behaviour.' For this reason, his advice to people who happen to be near someone who goes berserk is, 'Don't try to hold him down – back away! If you're not personally so threatened that you have to attack, he won't be so frightened that he has to fight back.'

Puffing on his pipe reflectively, as if nothing could ever disturb *his* equilibrium, Dr Ervin recalled some animal experiments. 'If you have a cat in a box, with a wire in his head,' he said, 'and you push a button that stimulates his amygdala, he will erect his hair, growl, fluff his tail, arch his back, put up his ears. He will look like a Hallowe'en cat, but he won't *do* anything, because there's nothing to do. This is to be understood as preparation for defence, for either fight or flight, as the situation dictates. But if there is an object present – a recently friendly cat or teddy bear, a large dog, anything, he will attack it in a very effective way. He will tear your hand to shreds if you don't have a glove on. On the other hand, if there is no target and he finds a panel that will open, he will flee and even move across hurdles to escape the stimulation. You have not really turned on aggression. There is interaction with his immediate environment to determine what happens next. There is *always* that interaction.'

What the stimulation does, then, is to arouse a pre-wired system in the brain which carries out acts of self-preservation. 'This anatomical circuit has been well worked out by physiologists,' said Dr Ervin. 'It can be called upon whenever the organism needs it. But in some cases it gets called upon erroneously, by electrical spikes that look like a signal to GO. Or else the damping, turn-off mechanism is somehow impaired.'

For in addition to the fight-or-flight system, there is another circuit in the brain that turns off such activity, Ervin explains. It is much less well explored, but it exists nevertheless. 'In the amygdala, it's very clear,' he says. 'The amygdaloid nucleus has two major parts, the old and the new. In the crocodile, a very primitive animal, there is almost no new amygdala. But in man there is very little of the old. In the cat or dog, it's about fifty-fifty, which makes them great research animals. If you stimulate the old portion of a cat's amygdala, you turn on preparation for fight or flight. But if you stimulate the new portion, the lateral part, the cat will purr, groom itself, present sexually and rub against your leg – it's a loving cat! Those two states seem to be mutually exclusive.'

This parallel 'system of tranquillity', as Dr Mark and Dr Ervin call it, is the basis of their optimism about the human lot. Man is not intrinsically destructive against his own species, they believe. Violence is not inevitable. There is an inborn mechanism to stop it, just as there is a mechanism to start it. The healthy brain can make a choice.

They claim to have evidence of this stopping mechanism in several of their patients, such as the engineer with several important patents to his credit, whom seven years of psychiatric treatment had not cured of terrible outbursts of violence. In his frenzy, he would sometimes pick up his wife and throw her against a wall. He had done this to her even when she was pregnant, and had attacked his children in the same way. After these fits of rage he would be overcome with remorse, begging his family's forgiveness. Finally, during one of his sessions with the psychiatrist, the doctor noticed that he was displaying the symptoms of a typical temporal-lobe seizure: staring, lip-smacking and salivation. Light dawned, and the engineer was referred to Massachusetts General Hospital, where tests showed that he suffered from epilepsy. Since no medication seemed to help him, the doctors decided on stereotactic surgery. In preparation for this, they implanted four strands of a dozen electrodes each and stimulated various points on both sides of his brain.

'I am losing control,' the engineer said suddenly when, unknown to him, an electrode stimulated a spot in the older part of his amygdala. His brow furrowed, and his eyes seemed hooded. 'Talking's difficult . . .' He complained of facial pain, similar to that which usually preceded his attacks. But as soon as Dr Mark switched to an electrode only four millimetres away, in the newer part of his amygdala, he relaxed visibly. 'I'm feeling in a good mood now,' he said, a smile slowly spreading on his face. He reported 'a feeling like Demerol . . . as though the room is getting larger and brighter . . . like I am floating on a cloud'. His facial pain disappeared within thirty seconds, though it usually lasted two to four hours. He became very talkative, and his happy mood continued for nearly a day after the current was turned off.

By stimulating the same spot in his 'system of tranquillity' every day, the doctors managed to keep the engineer free of rage for nearly three months. They could not go on stimulating him for the rest of his life, however, so eventually Dr Mark burned out the areas that seemed to cause trouble, in the old portions of the patient's left and right amygdalas. A burst of radio-frequency current, and the cells were destroyed. The engineer has never felt quite as happy as he did during his period of brain stimulation, but at least he has not had a single episode of rage since that time.

The team's surgery has had mixed results. Several patients have been free of violence for years after operations on both sides of their heads, but in others the attacks have recurred.

In his cluttered office Dr Ervin leaned back in his chair, puffed at his pipe, and tried to explain the team's work. A photograph of Einstein and the white pickled brain of a hydrocephalic kitten stared at him as he spoke. 'As I see the importance of our surgical cases,' he began, 'it is that during this limited historical period, when we have no better means for coping with these people's problem, they provide us with the only detailed insight we can get into the neural mechanism of the human brain.' If Dr Mark had not placed electrodes deep inside his patients' brains, for instance, he could never have recorded the abnormalities in their amygdalas, nor related them to their violent behaviour. Such precise information cannot be gathered from ordinary E E Gs on the surface of the head. The team hoped eventually to develop better methods of dealing with violence in epileptics, perhaps through chemicals. Such chemicals might be enclosed in tiny silicone membranes and implanted in the brain, to be released locally, in minute amounts, for years. Possibly hormone replacement in the brain might prove feasible.

Meanwhile, their work had led them to raise some interesting questions about the roots of violence in the general population. Since the limbic disorders they were treating seemed separate from their patients' epileptic seizures, the doctors began to wonder about violence in non-epileptics. What about the large numbers of people who regularly smash up their cars, fire their guns or assault their mates without having any of the traditional symptoms of epilepsy – did they, too, have some form of brain damage that might be corrected?

To find extreme cases of this sort, the team alerted the staffs of the emergency rooms at Massachusetts General Hospital and Boston City Hospital, asking them to send in any patients who felt they were losing control over aggressive impulses. Immediately they got two or three patients a day. 'It turned out to be one of the commonest complaints,' said Dr Ervin. One young man who appeared in the emergency room announced that he had just walked out, free from a grand jury hearing that had failed to indict him on a murder charge. 'But in fact, I did it, I killed my friend,' he blurted out. He'd nearly killed another man before, he said, and he was sure something terrible would happen again unless he got some help. The team gave him anti-seizure drugs, even though he had never had any overt epilepsy, plus tranquillizers and psychotherapy, and he is now under pretty good control. Another patient had tried to be admitted to the hospital eighteen times in the previous twenty months, whenever he had got into a fight and felt afraid he might kill somebody, but had been turned away every time because there were no facilities for people like him.

Soon the team had 134 self-referred patients to study – the kind of violent, unpredictable and dangerous people most doctors shun. Eight of them were murderers. Sixty per cent had at least one conviction for a crime of violence. And all of them admitted that they often used cars to relieve their tensions. One man had been stopped by the police for driving over 100 miles per hour at night without his lights on. To get even with any driver who cut in front of him, another habitually drove miles out of his way to force the other driver off the road.

Eventually, half of them were successfully treated with anti-convulsant drugs or tranquillizers, but not before they had scared the hospital staff out of its wits. Some nurses were so frightened that they threatened to quit, forcing the hospital administrator to insist that several of the most assaultive patients should be discharged. Meanwhile, the team was having trouble keeping the remaining patients in one place long enough to complete the three-day examinations – they would become restless and disappear, only to turn up again weeks or months later, after their next violent episode. To do a proper study, the doctors decided, they needed a captive population. The logical place was a federal prison, and there they went.

They were fascinated to discover that prisoners who were serving time for crimes of violence or sexual crimes were very similar to the outpatient group. 'They were generally poorer, dumber, older, more deprived and more alienated from the community's resources,' Dr Ervin said, 'but other than that there was little difference. They got involved in many brawls and beatings, they frequently lost control. You got the feeling that in most cases, if they had killed anyone, it was almost accidental – that they just happened to have a knife during one of their fights, or their opponent had hit his head too hard as he fell down. Most of them were distressed by it.' According to Dr Ervin, at least one quarter of the people arrested for crimes of this sort should be treated rather than locked up, because they have specific brain disease – conditions that might have been prevented, are now diagnosable, and can be treated, at least to some extent.

Detailed neurological and psychological examinations of eighty prisoners revealed either abnormal brain waves or symptoms of epilepsy in about half of the men tested. Since these recordings were made from the surface of the skull, the true proportion of abnormalities may have been even higher. A similar study showed that two thirds of the prisoners convicted of repeated personal assault in the Greater London area had abnormal brain waves emanating from areas deep behind the temples or in the upper brain stem. Possibly, if such people were given adequate treatment, large numbers of them might be released from prison – and prevented from further violence after their release.

This is exactly where problems arise, however. Are violent prisoners to be labelled 'brain-damaged' and subjected to brain surgery to cure them of violence? The mere idea of operating on people who have lost their freedom and doing irrevocable damage to their brains is horrifying, regardless of its possible benefits. Yet this was tried in 1968, in a prison hospital at Vacaville, California. Three prisoners with a history of episodic, uncontrollable violence had parts of their amygdalas destroyed by stereotactic surgery under the supervision of Dr Heimberger, who had pioneered the technique in the United States. According to prison officials, all three inmates and their families had consented to the operations. The results were uninspiring: one man, who originally showed marked improvement and was released on parole, ended right back in prison on a new robbery conviction and said he had begun to lose control of his emotions again. The second, in whom the operation has supposedly produced fair results, is still in jail. The third, who had shown little or no improvement, was eventually paroled. Nevertheless, some officials at the California Medical Facility in Vacaville wanted to continue the work, and in December 1971 the California Department of Corrections proposed an expanded programme of brain surgery for inmates with aggressive seizures caused by brain damage. As soon as this proposal became public, however, it created such an uproar that it was dropped. Instead, the department decided to limit its research programme to doing diagnoses and gathering data.

Dr Mark says that he is against brain operations for prisoners who suffer from temporal lobe epilepsy, even when psychotherapy and medicine fail, because 'informed consent is not possible in the prison setting at the present time'. Actual surgery is not the only danger, however. There is also the possibility that, by seeking ways to identify and screen people for 'episodic dyscontrol', justice officials may pick out all kinds of people, whose violence may have entirely different causes, and call them medical problems. Even in cases of temporal-lobe epilepsy, not all doctors agree that the violence is caused by the epilepsy. And without putting electrodes into a man's head, it is very difficult to make that diagnosis. So when law enforcement officials begin to look for an early-warning test that would identify the persons most likely to commit murder or violent crime because of brain damage, they are treading on extremely thin ice. Are people who make revolutions medical cases? Should their brains, too, be examined, or perhaps studied with electrodes?

In 1967 Dr Mark, Dr Sweet and Dr Ervin wrote a letter to the *Journal of the American Medical Association* that earned them enormous criticism. In it they suggested that the people who take violent part in urban riots may be suffering from focal brain damage. 'The real lesson of the urban rioting,' they concluded, 'is that, besides the need to study the social fabric that creates the riot atmosphere, we need intensive research and clinical studies of the individuals committing the violence. The goal of such studies would be to pinpoint, diagnose and treat those people with low violence thresholds before they contribute to further tragedies.' Since then, Dr Mark has partly changed his mind – he now feels that the police are often to blame for violence during riots – but he remains the target of demonstrations by young radicals at many of the scientific meetings he attends.

Dr Sweet recently commented about the surprising virulence of the attacks against him and his team. 'The criticism goes: "These fellows (my colleagues and I) may get so they *can* stop murderous behaviour in individuals. And we're afraid they will succeed, because then this information could be misused in other hands and lead to the performance of this kind of a pacification operation on those who are dissenting in society." Is this, then, a good reason for not seeking to learn how to control murderous behaviour in those individuals who have demonstrable organic brain disease?' he asked members of a conference on the physical manipulation of the brain sponsored by the Institute of Society, Ethics and the Life Sciences. Towards the end of the conference Dr Perry London, a professor of psychology and psychiatry at the University of Southern California, declared that 'the real issue is this: you have the capacity to go into this man's head, physically and directly. It is altogether plausible that doing so in an intelligent, careful way will permit you to directly ameliorate his behaviour. That capacity has absolutely nothing to do with epilepsy. It has absolutely nothing to do with an abnormal E E G. It's a simple technical fact. The man goes crazy. I'm talking now like a cop, or like a citizen who could get beat up, or like an aeroplane pilot who doesn't like people walking around with live grenades. The man goes crazy all the time. He is a terrible potential menace to society and to himself. You have a technology that permits you to address that directly. In less than five years Dr Delgado is going to make that technology so much easier that people without your sensibility and without your skill are going to be able to do that too. Then they're going to add two and two and get four, and say, "There's lots of people who act in lots of crazy ways and these doctors can't find anything wrong with their brain, their glands, or with their bodies; but they've tried every approach, like drugs and psychotherapy and so on and so forth, and none of these things have worked. Now these doctors have very safe, potentially very effective and very applicable techniques of going into the head. Why don't they do that?" That's what's going to happen.'

The trouble is that we have so few ways of dealing with violence, in criminals or others. We don't know how to cope with it or how to survive it; we certainly don't know how to prevent it. The problem is urgent, and people are clutching at straws. For the criminals themselves, the alternative to treatment (which doesn't always work) may be a lifetime spent behind bars. (Someday soon, said Robert Livingston, Professor of Neurosciences at the University of California at San Diego, we may look back on our present treatment of prisoners and find it barbaric – as brutal as that of the epileptics and mentally ill 'who, in the history of our own country, were imprisoned and flogged for their own good and that of society, and with full sanction of medical and religious leadership'. Instead of our self-defeating penal system, he proposes 'proper intervention' in the brains of prisoners who have temporal-lobe defects.) For other people who suffer from such attacks of violence, the alternative is a nightmarish existence over which they have no control. Better techniques and much research are sorely needed. But meanwhile, what should one do?

'I follow a simple prescription, generally, for deciding on all elective medical procedures,' Dr Paul MacLean told a meeting of the National Institutes of Health on brain surgery recently. 'First I ask, is this a procedure I would want done to a friend? If the answer is yes, I ask myself, is this a procedure I would want done to a member of my family – my mother, my wife, my child? And if the answer is still yes, I ask, is this something I would want done to myself?' Thereupon he asked the audience for a show of hands from all those who were willing to have electrodes implanted in their amygdala. Not one hand was raised.

10 Where are they going?

The brain changes that are possible today are just a small beginning.

Only a few generations of scientists have dared to explore the human brain. It's only twenty years since the first burst of discoveries in the neurosciences revealed the existence of pain and pleasure centres, the significance of the corpus callosum, a few clues to memory and some physical effects of experience.

For a while, during that time, brain research was the scene of a sort of gold rush, where anybody armed with the equivalent of a mere pick and shovel had a chance to make a fabulous find. But it soon became clear that things weren't quite that simple. The brain contained more intricate and secret codes than man had ever dreamed of in his philosophy – layers upon layers of mysteries, hidden springs and triggers countered by complex mechanisms for blocking. No individual scientist could begin to understand them. No scientific discipline could even point the way.

Realizing that they needed to combine their disparate skills, the brain researchers have regrouped. Chemists, biologists, anatomists, physiologists, surgeons, psychiatrists, psychologists, computer technicians, engineers and dozens of sophisticated hybrids are now converging on the brain with new techniques and new tools. In the near future, some spectacular discoveries may be expected.

Where will they take us? At the very least, they will prevent a great deal of misery – from mental illnesses that existing treatments cannot cure, from memory loss, insomnia, certain kinds of mental retardation and other ills. They are also opening up staggering possibilities for the enhancement of human life, for greater understanding and more self-control. But as I worked on this book, I kept running into examples of how even the crude brain operations and chemical treatments that are known today can be abused. There was a glaring gap between the people who did the research and those who used its fallout sometimes recklessly. In addition, there were some disturbing implications about the research itself. I found myself alternately excited and appalled.

It was exciting to learn, in Ross Adey's Space Biology Lab, that the brain speaks, through brain waves, and that some of its language can be understood with the aid of computers. It would be good to be able to tune into a pilot's brain wave, to know when he is in the right state of mind to land a plane properly, and to avoid the kind of crashes attributable to 'human error'. Such mind-reading – or prophecy – might also give many children the satisfaction of errorless learning. But what would happen to my privacy if someone could tell whether I was planning to say 'yes' or 'no' even a fraction of a second before I said it?

Furthermore, as soon as one gains the power to recognize certain brain states, there is a temptation to change or control them. It's wonderful that the new techniques of bio-feedback may enable us to control our own brain waves as efficiently as if we were yogis. I found it a most enticing possibility. On the other hand, what about the power of electrical stimulation to change both brain states and behaviour? Or the pharmacologists' demonstrations of how easily brain states can be changed with drugs?

I could admire Dr Delgado's new double-barrelled gadget, the dialytrode, which stood ready to send either chemical or electrical stimulation to any point in the brain – but I hated to think of how it might be used. Logically, this work had to lead to putting implants deep into a person's brain, either temporarily or permanently. Dr Delgado's experiments with the chimpanzee Paddy showed that such implants could be controlled by a distant computer. Eventually, the computer itself might be enclosed in the brain, together with the electrodes, to regulate a person's conduct in a wholly invisible way.

Dr Old's finding that there exists 'a river of reward' in the brain also lends itself to strange speculations. Naturally, writers of science fiction have had a field day with descriptions of entire populations stimulating themselves in the brain, through implanted electrodes, to obtain a pleasure greater than sex. For psychologists, however, his finding was a happy one, since it showed that people's actions are prompted not only by the need to reduce painful drives, but also by the possibility of pleasure or joy. That is how we learn, they concluded – by a natural activation of our pleasure centres when we do things right. Of course I welcomed this idea. But I lost some of my enthusiasm when I discovered that an efficient way to make animals perform certain tasks – now the standard procedure in many labs – is to insert electrodes into their brains' pleasure areas and reward them with stimulation at chosen times. Apparently none can resist that kind of Skinnerian shaping.

Each kind of brain change has its hopeful and its alarming aspects. Take the control of memory – what would happen if 'memory pills' suddenly became available, together with drugs to obliterate experience? Right now, doctors are free to give any young child powerful mind-changing drugs simply because his teachers or parents find him 'hyperactive'; in some cases the drugs may be fully justified and helpful, but in other cases not. In mental hospitals and nursing homes, tranquillizers are forced down the throats of patients, mostly for the convenience of the staff. What kind of abuses may be expected after the development of even more varied and potent drugs? Clearly some safeguards should be built in ahead of time.

I became aware of the need for safeguards even in attempts to help the crippled and the blind. Normally one would consider all such efforts unquestionably worthwhile – but not if they involve the brain. Here one cannot forget the possibility that the new techniques may someday be misused, though of course their value to the handicapped may prove immense.

Suppose you were totally blind, but could be made to see through a brain operation. Would you agree to having it performed? Most blind people, apparently, would not. They might eagerly ask for the most delicate or painful operation on their eyes, provided it stopped just short of the grey matter inside their skull. An audience of blind persons in Ohio listened with great interest as a lecturer told them about seeing-aids that use TV cameras to activate tiny tactile stimulators placed on the forehead or the back so as to provide cues about nearby objects. But they recoiled when he described the work of a British physiologist, Dr Giles Brindley of the University of London and Maudsley Hospital, who had similar stimulators inserted directly into a patient's head.

The stalwart patient who volunteered for this operation was a fifty-two-year-old woman, a nurse who had recently lost her sight. She still wears the handmade device that Dr Brindley and a surgeon inserted into her head in 1967. It is a fairly small, curved packet of eighty electrodes placed on her right visual cortex, at the back of her brain, and connected by wire to a large shell of radio receivers, about a third of an inch thick and as wide as a man's hand, implanted over her skull but under her scalp. The receivers are activated by an even larger skull-cap containing radio transmitters, which the nurse can put on her head. When these are turned on, she sees thirty-seven little specks of light, similar to the 'stars' people experience when they bump their heads in the dark. Some of the specks are tiny, some are elongated 'like a matchstick at arm's length', others are round and cloudlike. Although most of the experts said the system would never work, these thirty-seven 'phosphenes' do produce patterns that the nurse can identify, somewhat like the lights on a theatre façade, depending on which electrodes have been activated.

In theory, then, if many more electrodes were placed in a blind person's visual cortex, he might learn to distinguish shapes and even letters. A modified TV camera would be required to translate these shapes into dots and then transmit them by radio to his brain. Someday, this camera might be made to fit directly into the person's eye, and even connect with his ocular muscles. Artificial eyes that move – although they do nothing else – already exist, for cosmetic use; they could be adapted for this purpose. So far Dr Brindley's device has been of no use to the nurse, but more advanced models may eventually help blind people to read and get about, seeing one shape at a time as if through an enormous magnifying glass.

While Dr Brindley worked on the blind, a scientist of the Stanford Research Institute, in California, began an equally startling, though potentially useful project to help the paralysed. Dr Lawrence Pinneo hoped that stroke victims might make their own limbs move by directing a computer to stimulate electrodes implanted in their brains. He wanted to take advantage of the fact that large quantities of healthy nerves and tissue remain under a damaged cortex, particularly in the brain stem, where many motor commands from the cortex are normally integrated. After mapping the brains of several hundred squirrel and rhesus monkeys, he learned which centres in the brain stem control such movements as bending a paw, foreleg or hip. (Though each of these movements appears simple, it may involve the co-ordination of as many as thirty different muscles.) He placed electrodes in these centres, and tried to stimulate them in specific sequences.

Films of his research show an anaesthetized monkey lying limply in a sort of hammock, its arms and legs dangling down the hammock's sides. As the electrodes in its brain stem receive current, the monkey's limbs straighten out and start to move – first one leg, then the other, in a running motion. Then all four limbs move, as if the monkey were preparing to jump. All this happens while the animal remains profoundly asleep.

Since he could not find a monkey that had suffered a stroke, Dr Pinneo decided to produce similar damage surgically. He removed part of the cortex of a rhesus monkey, paralysing its right arm. Next he inserted electrodes into its brain stem and programmed thirteen of these electrodes in different sequences, to be run with the aid of a computer. One sequence allowed him to make the monkey's paralysed arm reach for food, grasp it and put it into its mouth; another sequence had the monkey reaching out and up, as if to climb a bar; a third made it reach backward to scratch its tail. Finally the monkey was placed next to a switch on the computer. It took only one trial to teach the animal to press the switch with its good hand, enabling it to use the paralysed arm to reach and pick up food.

If similar systems were ready for use on human beings, some people might want them, just as cardiac patients now gladly accept having electric pacemakers inserted into their hearts. Dr Pinneo hopes to be able to continue his work along these lines, although he realizes that it might eventually present some problems. 'It's quite true that if I succeed in controlling the limb movements of a paralysed person, I could also do it with someone who is not paralysed,' he said. 'I think brain research needs to be monitored, and each project evaluated on its own merits.' If anyone tried to push his kind of research beyond its therapeutic applications, he believes it should be stopped.

For the moment, brain implants remain thoroughly impractical. 'The electrodes that exist today cannot be implanted for a long time without damage,' said Dr Karl Frank, a neurophysiologist who directs a major effort in the National Institutes of Health to develop better aids for the blind, the paralysed and people with other neurological handicaps. 'People who say otherwise aren't bothering to look at what damage they actually produce.' Electrodes are cemented to the skull, and they are rigid, he explains. If the patient is quiet, the electrodes remain stationary with respect to the soft mass of his brain. If he moves suddenly in a straight line, his brain will move slightly with respect to the electrodes, though probably not enough to do much harm. But if he's subjected to rotational acceleration, as in whiplash, his brain will lag behind his skull. 'In that case, an electrode which is rigidly affixed to the skull ploughs through the brain, just as a spoon fixed to a bowl would cut through a bowlful of jelly,' Dr Frank said. 'So we need an electrode that's flexible and moves with the brain. We don't have anything I'd be willing to put in a human now, other than for diagnosis which is necessary because of epilepsy or some other problem.' Even if flexible electrodes are developed, no one yet knows how to prevent damage from the complex electrochemical reactions that sometimes occur, over a period of time, between the electrodes and the surrounding fluids in the brain. There is also the danger that scar tissue around the electrodes might itself produce epileptic seizures.

However, someday the technical difficulties may be overcome, or perhaps brain stimulation will be possible without surgically entering the skull. And then the real problems will begin. For the easier and safer a procedure, the more casually people use it, and the more likely that it will be abused – as has already happened with drugs.

If so, if their findings are used improperly, the brain scientists cannot be held directly responsible. It would be unfair to blame them for our present epidemic of drug abuse, for instance. They might have done more to explain the dangers of certain drugs, but it is not their fault that addiction is spreading. Nor did they ever intend that tranquillizers should be used to drug people into a stupor.

The brain researchers' ultimate goal is far removed from such behaviour control. As in any fledgling science, they are forced to work somewhat haphazardly, like children exploring a new toy. They try this or that, just to see how the brain works, since there is still no theory to explain even a fraction of the brain's operations. Other than curiosity, what drives them is, first of all, the thought that they may learn to cure some of the mental diseases that now afflict millions of people, and prevent all kinds of other miseries. Even this would not fully satisfy many of them, however. The really exciting part of their work is the much more revolutionary possibility that they could extend human abilities *beyond* the normal, or at least beyond what is considered normal today.

That's what the future of brain research is all about. Bringing people closer to 'normality' may be laudable and useful and what pays the rent, but actually the brain is man's last frontier – so why stop there?

Just as the invention of clothing made it possible and 'normal' for human beings to live in a wide range of climates, and machines have extended the power of man's muscles, other products of the human brain can now extend man's potential in different ways. And here I must share some of the brain-changers' optimism.

Within a few decades, they may know how to make babies become more intelligent and emotionally stable, as well as more peaceful. At present, their information is still extremely sketchy. But several findings could be combined, to multiply their effects. The Berkeley experiments which showed that changing the toys in a rat nursery school every day produced increases in the rats' cortical weight fit in well with Seymour Levine's demonstration that variety in the environment can promote emotional stability. The work on the damaging effects of lead poisoning and other kinds of pollution could be linked with research on the brain's critical need for proteins in infancy. Victor Denenberg's finding that mothering by a peaceful rat 'aunt' during a critical period immediately after birth will prevent mice of a highly aggressive strain from fighting each other at maturity agrees with the notion that certain levels of expectancy are built in and fixed in earliest infancy. If one could set these levels deliberately, so that the fight-or-flight response is aroused as seldom as possible, future generations might be much more peaceful than those of today. Possibly drugs could enhance both these processes – the growth of the cortex as the baby learns to deal with more variety, and the maintenance of emotional stability.

Scientists have already succeeded in teaching fish to spawn in specific streams by imprinting the odour of these streams on baby fish as soon as they are hatched. Who knows how many other kinds of imprinting can be devised for human infants, to make them thirst for knowledge, for peace, or for love of others, in later years?

We are only beginning to understand the power of such interventions. Even today, children who are born of affluent, educated parents have an enormous advantage over other children because of the way they are brought up. There can be no equality of opportunity until we are able to reproduce such circumstances for any child, beginning at the moment of conception. The brain scientists hope that they will not only achieve such equality, but will find ways in which children of any social class can be developed far beyond what they are today.

Researchers may have even more exciting contributions to make at the other end of man's life span. Why should people lose their memories and their intellectual powers as they age? It may be 'normal', but it is certainly not necessary, and it makes a mockery of the extra years they have gained from better medical care.

The number of people over sixty-five has been increasing far more rapidly than the general population throughout the Western world. The number of people over seventy-five is growing most rapidly, with the centenarians – of whom there are now thirteen thousand in the United States – increasing most of all. Until recently, psychologists made the mistake of assuming that intelligence automatically declined with age. They were misled because they tested cross-sections of people, and the older groups had received less education than the younger ones. When they began to do longitudinal studies that followed certain persons over a period of time, they discovered that most people *gained*, rather than lost in intelligence, right through their fifth decade of life. The only thing their subjects lost, after the age of sixty, was speed, especially on motor tasks. Otherwise, the most striking feature of old people's scores on intelligence tests was their stability until the age of seventy-three.

When intelligence did decline, it was usually in the presence of disease. While studying aged twins who had been followed up for several decades, Dr Lissy Jarvik and her associates at the New York State Psychiatric Institute discovered that the twins whose scores went down tended to die within the next five years.

At the time of the test, these twins did not appear to be ill and medical tests showed nothing wrong. Possibly the psychological tests picked up minute changes in brain functioning caused by an inadequate blood supply to the brain resulting from arteriosclerosis or other ills.

If such decline is not taken for granted, perhaps it can be stopped or reversed, preventing the terrible spiral into senility that afflicts so many thousands of old people. Senility means far more than a loss of memory, although that is a prominent feature. Senile people are also incontinent, confused, disoriented, generally debilitated, and depressed. Since they cannot live alone, they are often 'warehoused' in dismal nursing homes or in the back wards of mental hospitals. Yet many of them, who are basically depressed, could be given anti-depressant drugs. Another large group actually suffers from the delayed effect of hypertension – even a moderate degree of hypertension can severely impair one's brain unless treatment is started in time. Others, whose memory is gone, might benefit enormously from memory drugs such as those now being developed by Dr James McGaugh.

Even 'normal' old people, who seem alert and intelligent, often complain bitterly about their loss of memory. Recently Dr Jarvik discovered that this may be related to chromosomal damage. She found that the aged twins who did poorly on memory tests had a loss of chromosomes in many of their white blood cells, which meant that other dividing cell systems in their bodies, including their brain's glial cells, were probably damaged in a similar way. Such damage could certainly interfere with mental functioning. The few eighty-five-year-olds in her study who did not have such chromosome loss still scored well on memory tests. No one yet knows whether the chromosome loss actually causes forgetfulness or, if so, how to prevent or retard it; but at least Dr Jarvik feels she now has a good tool – the study of chromosomes in white blood cells – with which to study age changes and perhaps evaluate new treatments that are proposed to help the aged. For example, some senile patients have appeared rejuvenated after treatments in a high-pressure oxygen chamber. She believes that within the next ten years scientists will have effective means of preventing both the forgetfulness of the aged and true senility.

Eventually, special programmes of brain hygiene might be developed to sharpen people's mental faculties at every stage of life. Before reaching one's sixties, for instance, one might undertake a regimen involving a variety of brain-stretching activities, food supplements, special diets or drugs to control even low levels of hypertension, memory drugs, oxygen treatments or various kinds of bio-feedback training. These would be followed by annual psychological check-ups (which would become as common as physical check-ups are today) to detect any sign of mental deterioration and fight it with specific remedies. Millions of aged people would then be able to retain their full mental powers and their memories to the end – assuming they had access to such programmes. At least the brain scientists would have made it possible for us to control our own intellectual futures. And with continuing advances in longevity, we might gain as much as twenty or thirty years of full, adult intellectual vigour.

The brain scientists' goal of extending human abilities will be reached only when they find ways of linking, and thus amplifying, the many new techniques now being developed. In scattered laboratories, and in the minds of many researchers, are new findings that could, for example, vastly improve learning speed and efficiency at any age. But there is no unifying theory. There are only seeds of the progress to come.

Suppose it were proved that exposing one's head to a field of magnetic radiation in the theta range did help one to learn rapidly and well, as Rochelle Gavalas's experiments imply, and that this were perfectly safe. Suppose one also had access to a computer that presented new information, or new problems, only when one's brain waves were at their most receptive state, so that one never made any errors. Suppose further that one could train oneself, through bio-feedback, to produce at will the best kind of brain waves for learning. Or that safe and effective memory pills were at hand. Any combination of these could turn an average person into a super-learner, who advanced by leaps and bounds across any subject he pleased and remembered it permanently. The cumulative effect of such learning might be tremendous.

Similarly, a combination of bio-feedback training with drugs and, perhaps, exposure to certain magnetic fields might make people sleep so profoundly and so well that a couple of hours' sleep a night would be sufficient, and a few minutes' nap in the middle of the day could recharge them with fresh energy and zest.

Some other possible combinations sound suspiciously like science fiction. The scientists who mentioned them know they are quite far-fetched, but find them worth considering. By using the new technology of brain implants together with certain powerful tools, for instance, it might become feasible to extend man's senses beyond the five he was born with. A human brain might be linked directly to a computer, a microscope or an x-ray camera. The information from these instruments would be radioed to an array of implanted electrodes which might at first produce meaningless patterns, but which one might learn to interpret. In effect, one might become like Superman.

'Would you really like to have this done to you?' I asked Dr Frank of the National Institutes of Health, when he mentioned the possibility of such brain implants. 'If it were safe? Of course!' he replied. 'Wouldn't you? I'm going to sail across the Atlantic this summer [he pointed to a picture of a sailboat on his wall]. Wouldn't you like to go to the moon? There is some danger in crossing the street to get to the other side. You've got to balance the small risk against the small gain. It's people who make *wrong* compromises with risk who live foolishly.'

'It won't happen in our lifetime,' he added. 'But if you give people golden tools like these, they'll keep putting them together – you can't stop them! Assuming, of course, that electrodes can be so developed that they don't do any harm. It will probably happen so gradually that people will scarcely notice it happening. They'll think they knew about it all along.'

Another way to help our brains along might be through genetics – or so suggests Dr Robert Sinsheimer, of the California Institute of Technology, who thinks that future generations will see us rather as we see Winnie-the-Pooh, the bear of very little brain: 'Frail and slow in logic, weak in memory and pale in abstraction, but . . . on occasions possessed of innate common sense and uncommon perception'. He chafes at our present limitations. Our brains are limited in speed, compared to computers, he complains. They are limited in the number of things they can attend to simultaneously; limited in their ability to communicate, especially to communicate feelings or emotions; and limited in the kind of concepts they can formulate. 'What else can we sensibly expect, when we are apparently the first creatures with any significant capacity for abstract thought?' he asks. Yet it may still be possible for man to improve his own brain. Though this is clearly a bootstrap project, it is what we have done all the way from the jungle.

In time, we may be able to define just how man's genes differ from those of the monkey; quantitatively, there is very little difference. By reproducing this evolutionary leap in the laboratory, we might gain some clues to the next big leap forward. And we might find that an exceedingly small genetic change would have enormous consequences. It might, for example, 'expand consciousness into unknown sensations and into undreamt-of intensities,' says Dr Sinsheimer. 'If this sounds absurd, consider that many vertebrates have no colour vision at all. By changing their genetic programme, an entire new sense has been added.' A few strategically placed genetic alterations might allow human beings to turn off pain, enter new mental states or push back their present intellectual and conceptual limits.

Nothing seems impossible, if one works through the brain. And most of the proposed changes appear to be for the good.

Yet the prospect of some human beings having so much power over the brains of others is enough to send shivers down one's spine.

The enthusiasm and recklessness with which leucotomies were performed during the 1930s and 1940s do not inspire confidence in existing safeguards. Many of the operation's drawbacks did not become apparent until it was too late. After leucotomy, patients were certainly less anxious, but when they returned to their families, their relatives found them totally changed: unfeeling, gross, unable to plan for the future. 'He doesn't have a soul any more,' complained some of the wives of patients. Roughly 10 per cent of the patients became epileptic years later, because of scar tissue from the operation. Yet for a decade leucotomies were so widely accepted that even G.P.s could perform them almost freehand, with what were sarcastically called 'ice pick' techniques. To this day, mutilating operations continue to be performed on various parts of the brain, especially in Britain where restricted leucotomies remained popular long after their use had declined elsewhere. Even though the techniques are more precise and the brain destruction is more limited, the results of such operations are still highly uncertain.

Nor have drugs companies given us much reason to believe that they will voluntarily refrain from misleading advertisements – particularly about drugs to relieve anxiety, insomnia, depression and the like. By now, half of the population of the United States uses mind-changing drugs occasionally, and 17 per cent of adults use them frequently. Physicians have crossed the boundaries of traditional medical care. As a result every deviant behaviour – alcoholism, drug addiction, 'hyperactivity' – can now be regarded as an illness, in the hope of curing it. But 'if alcoholism is defined as a disease, it can be treated by psychosurgery,' points out Dr Herbert Vaughan, a neurologist at the Einstein College of Medicine. So can violent behaviour (however justifiable), homosexuality or any socially unacceptable trait. The dangers of this tendency should be obvious to

221

anyone familiar with the Russian practice of calling political dissidents mentally ill and then locking them up in institutions where they are forced to undergo stultifying drug treatments.

The tendency to prescribe drugs for social, rather than medical, uses is spreading, however, and it is becoming more respectable. Not long ago, Dr Kenneth Clark proposed that 'scientific biochemical intervention' should be used to reduce man's barbaric instincts. All the world leaders should be given peace pills, he said. (This led the *New Yorker* to wonder, 'Who is to be our President's pusher? Who will decide when to administer the drug and when to withhold it? Who will administer the dose?') Even so conservative a group as the National Education Association predicted that, by the late 1970s, 'school faculties will include biochemical therapist-pharmacists, whose services will increase as biochemical therapy and memory-improvement chemicals are introduced more widely.'

The government agencies that pass on most grants for brain research have been generally conservative and prudent. So have the majority of brain scientists. But out where people have to deal with urgent practical problems, there is strong pressure to use any technique or any drug at hand, regardless of its risks or how little is known about it. That is where the danger lies.

The basic questions are, Who will do what to whom? And who will decide? Brain changes that are made voluntarily, in one's own brain – through bio-feedback, other forms of self-discipline, or drugs – are obviously in a different class from two other kinds: (1) changes made under independent contract, as in psychotherapy, in which the patient is a party to the treatment and wants it, but is free to leave at any time; and (2) changes imposed on a dependent group that has no voice in the matter – for example, drugs administered to patients in mental hospitals or in nursing homes to keep them quiet. These three categories require entirely different safeguards.

Suppose the brain scientists find the perfect aphrodisiac, or a harmless and non-addictive 'soma', as in *Brave New World*. Why should anyone intervene in its use by adults? Similarly, I can't imagine any restrictions on the use of yoga, Zen, bio-feed-back, or other methods of changing one's brain states through learning. Of course, some addictive drugs are prohibited or re-quire a doctor's prescription. On the theory that society has the responsibility to prevent people from committing suicide, or at least to try to prevent it, I welcome these minor restrictions on my freedom. But non-addictive drugs such as marijuana must sooner or later be legalized, joining the more addictive tobacco and alcohol on the psychological bill of fare, together with coffee and tea. The nation's 'pharmacological Calvinism' is undergoing a rapid erosion, according to Dr Gerald Klerman, a professor of psychiatry at Harvard. He sees us headed towards some kind of 'psychotropic hedonism', in which we will be free to choose between drugs to enhance our performance, drugs to help us learn and remember better, drugs to stimulate or calm us and a variety of drugs to increase our pleasure – all without fear of permanent damage by chemicals.

The moment one leaves this category of voluntary brain changes and asks a doctor or surgeon to do something to one's brain, however, the situation changes radically. 'There are no legal controls on psychosurgery,' Dr Vaughan commented, 'no safeguards at the present time except the conscience of the physician . . . It is a strictly *laissez faire*, entrepreneurial rela-tionship.' He finds it scandalous that we have no better report-ing on such cases. Nobody even knows how many brain opera-tions are being performed on people to change their behaviour (as opposed to removing brain tumours or doing other essential surgery), although the figure has been estimated at around 500 a year in Britain and almost as many in the U S. The late appears to be growing. Nor does anyone have figures on shock treatments, which some institutions dish out in horrifyingly large doses, up to seventy or even 200 treatments for a single person, when the accepted limit is ten to twenty. Dr Vaughan believes that a national registry should be set up to keep records on all psychosurgery, as is now done to keep track of heart trans-plants.

Doctors notoriously protect one another. Medical societies refuse to take any action unless the patient himself files a formal complaint, at which point the worst they can do is to dismiss the doctor from membership. Yet patients are seldom able to do so. A person who has become addicted to barbiturates or amphetamines is usually so dependent on the doctor who prescribes them that he would never dare testify against him. After long series of shock treatments, patients tend to lose their memory. And although surgeons sometimes say that none of their lobotomized patients has ever complained, what is left of these patients? Who is there to complain?

Unfortunately, doctors sometimes do not know any other way to cope with totally intractable cases – for example, patients so self-destructive that when not restrained they bite their own flesh off. The decision to operate on a person's brain because of his behaviour should not be left entirely in the hands of an individual physician, however. The results of such operations can be too far-reaching for the responsibility to be placed on any one person. Some kind of control must be exerted beforehand.

In the United States, surgeons do not need the approval of any other doctor before launching into psychosurgery – not even when dealing with the brains of children. A Mississippi surgeon, Dr Orlando J. Andy, has operated on children as young as six – most of them institutionalized children – who were referred to him for such loosely defined behaviour problems as 'erratic aggression', 'hyper-reactivity' and 'emotional instability'. He cut the brain of an epileptic nine-year-old boy five times, destroying more of the boy's thalamus, a central part of the brain that is deeply involved in emotion, four of these times, because the boy was 'hyperactive, combative, explosive, destructive, sadistic'. In between, he cut another brain structure, the fornix. After the fifth operation, the boy's behaviour was finally 'improved' – though he deteriorated intellectually. Dr Andy explains that such operations are necessary 'for custodial purposes, when patients require inordinate amounts of care.' Yet almost nothing is known about the effects of these operations.

There should be a Bill of Rights to protect the brains of children, even when their parents sign a so-called 'informed consent'. Such consent may be totally meaningless. Who gave the parents the information? This cannot be left to the person who wishes to perform the operation. Did the institution pressure them to agree? Was there anyone in authority to whom they might have appealed?

When leucotomies were in vogue in the 1940s, they were inflicted mostly on schizophrenic patients in the back wards of state hospitals – a dependent group that was thoroughly defenceless. Even there, the largest number of operations was performed on the most vulnerable: the poor, the blacks and women, according to Dr Peter Breggin, a psychoanalyst and novelist of Washington, DC, who has been leading a one-man crusade against all forms of psychosurgery.

Clearly, the least powerful groups stand the greatest risk – and need the most protection against brain-changing techniques. Thus not only children, but also adult prisoners, the mentally ill, the mentally retarded, and the aged in nursing homes need a Bill of Rights, or at least some kind of buffer between their brains and the managers of desperately understaffed institutions, who may be tempted to try anything that will make their charges more manageable. Lacking such a buffer, these dependent people find their identity directly threatened by treatments no longer aimed at curing an individual patient, but at silencing troublesome groups. And it doesn't take much paranoia in such circumstances to see impending political plots – against blacks, leftists, women or any other section of the population.

Just because brain surgery arouses so much revulsion, however, it is less likely to be abused on a large scale than drugs or other means of control. Anything that involves penetrating the skull and manipulating the brain produces horror. It violates a basic taboo – some researchers call it the 'skull barrier'. 'People sort of treasure this piece of skull,' said one scientist sarcastically. 'They consider it sacred.' When news of psychosurgery in a California prison leaked out, there was such a public outcry that the programme was immediately stopped (after a total of three operations), with little prospect of starting again. Besides, psychosurgery is expensive and requires highly trained surgeons. It is much easier to use drugs.

With drugs, the danger is so insidious that researchers who have given the matter some thought, such as Dr Willard Gaylin of the Institute of Society, Ethics and the Life Sciences, actually welcome the controversy now surrounding psychosurgery. They see it serving as a sort of focus, bringing attention to the subtle but larger problems arising from all forms of coercion under the guise of mental health.

No 'informed consent' is required when an institutionalized patient or prisoner is given drugs. Consent is necessary only when such people take part in research projects, as often happens, particularly in prisons in America, since American drug companies cannot find any better or cheaper guinea-pigs anywhere: the going rate of pay is one dollar a day. Most prisoners are eager to receive this pittance, having no other source of funds. The managers of the institutions that allow such programmes may also receive various benefits from the drug companies. But the consent forms that the prisoners are asked to sign are often a farce. Recently a law professor asked for details about some 'behavioural control' experiments being run in a Maryland prison with new drugs. 'Does he understand the effects of the drug?' the professor asked about one inmate who received doses of a female hormone. 'Yes, we explained the whole thing to him,' the director of the prison replied, 'we don't want any misunderstanding.' 'Well,' the professor continued, 'what are the effects?' 'We don't know,' he was told; 'that's what they're trying to find out.' Just as with psychosurgery, then, there is an urgent need for some kind of ombudsman or buffer to stand between dependent groups and the people who have the power to give them mind-changing drugs.

Some national standards will have to be set regarding the use of either psychosurgery or drugs for social control. Neither physicians nor brain scientists are the keepers of our moral values. Before any decisions are made affecting children, for instance – before some 200,000 schoolchildren with behaviour problems are given amphetamines or other drugs to reduce their 'hyperactivity' – there should be public hearings and broad discussions, especially by school boards and parents. There should be guidelines set by reputable national bodies that include a cross-section of the public, not just the scientific or medical establishments. There should be much more widespread interest and concern.

Another cause for concern is the recent proliferation of behaviour modification treatments. Patients who have annoying traits may be conditioned to change their behaviour by psychologists who give them mild electric shocks from a portable shocker every time they misbehave – somewhat like a dog being whipped by its trainer. Crude as this may be, it appears quite effective for specific kinds of behaviour. But the mind boggles at what might happen if the sensitive and high-speed technology of bio-feedback were linked to such punishment.

As scientists offer society more and more techniques for the control of human minds, it will become increasingly important to make informed decisions on how to use them. In each case this will require tackling some troublesome issues:

1. How reversible is the proposed treatment? That is often far from clear. Even one session of L S D therapy, coupled with suggestion, may irrevocably change a person's orientation to life. With or without benefit of chemicals, psychotherapy can also produce deep changes in one's personality, changes that might be reversed only at great cost. Psychology students who volunteer for psychological experiments may be totally shattered by the revelation of their own inadequacy, especially if they are publicly ridiculed. (A few such students have committed suicide.) Prisoners who are forced to take part in encounter therapy sometimes find it equally destructive. And brain changes resulting from alterations in one's earliest environment can never be totally wiped out.

Some drug effects are temporary; others leave lasting marks.

Most addictions are permanent. If taken over a long period of time, the chemical treatments for certain kinds of mental illness may produce irreversible brain damage.

Electrical stimulation of the brain is essentially reversible, but its effects may last a long time. And if it were used to reinforce certain kinds of learning, its results might never be unlearned. However, the most irreversible changes of all are clearly those resulting from the surgical destruction of part of one's brain.

2. How would it affect the individual's identity? At first glance, invading the brain with implanted electrodes seems one of the worst possible threats to one's identity. But would an epileptic really be better off with repeated, incapacitating epileptic fits than with a painless brain implant that stopped such seizures before they started? The fits might be a far greater threat to his true identity. (And if neither alternative seemed bearable, would it be preferable to split his corpus callosum and have him acquire, in effect, *two* separate identities?)

On the other hand, implants designed to change a person's behaviour, to reward or punish certain states of mind selectively, would totally destroy his autonomy. So would drugs administered to a person just to make him more manageable.

3. How would it affect civil liberties? This involves finding out which groups would be the most likely targets of the proposed treatment, and why.

4. What might be its unintended effects? This is perhaps the most difficult question of all. Brain-changing techniques lend themselves to the most unlikely uses. In France, where generations of peasant women have painstakingly force-fed geese by hand (to fatten their livers for good *foie gras*), surgeons have begun to take over the job, performing a delicate operation on the animals' hypothalamus to knock out their centres of satiety. This makes the geese eat incessantly – as if of their own free will – damaging their insides and consuming almost as much as when they were stuffed by hand. To top it all, a drug company

is now developing a chemical that could be injected directly into the animals' brains to produce the same effect in only a few minutes, at negligible cost.

There is something particularly revolting about these self-stuffing geese. Surely the American scientists who investigated the brain mechanisms responsible for appetite and satiety could not foresee such applications of their work. It makes one wonder how our own brains may be changed someday, and for whose benefit. What may all this research do to human beings – inadvertently?

The brain scientists themselves are worried about this. There has been much soul-searching in the big universities and world capitals where scientists now meet for discussions about the ethics of their work. There is talk of calling a moratorium on certain kinds of brain research. There is a movement for the adoption of a new Hippocratic oath for the life sciences. For the past decade, students have flocked into the neurosciences from other fields such as physics in the belief, as Professor Hans-Lukas Teuber of MIT put it, that 'this is still one area to which people can turn when they don't want to build weapons'. But after some exposure to the research now going on, some of the best young scientists begin to have doubts: they suspect that this, too, might be used for evil ends. A few drop out or become militants. To create a better climate for all workers in this field, Dr Teuber has proposed that young brain scientists, like young physicians, should be required to swear that they will never participate in any project that might be harmful to men.

Good intentions alone are not enough to guard against the unintended results of their work, however. Probably people of widely differing backgrounds, including economists, philosophers and practical politicians, would be in a better position to foresee such consequences than the brain scientists. What is needed, then, is some sort of watchdog committee that would alert the public to possible applications of the new findings as they appear, and a framework through which the nation can reach wise decisions on what to allow and what to stop. It is essential that such a framework should be developed *before* new advances in technology make the procedures so easy that almost anyone can use them.

Experts are 'notorious order-takers', Professor David Krech stated. They can provide facts, but not decisions. Like an ancient prophet, he urges us to prepare to deal with the difficult moral issues that face us today, and those that will arise in the future. Even the idea of brain transplants, which seemed utterly improbable a few years ago, is beginning to sound more feasible every day; 'We may yet live to see it,' he said. The question then would be, who is the donor? Who the recipient? What is the identity of the creature produced by such surgery? 'We all suffer from a lack of imagination,' Dr Krech warned. 'I try to be as far out as I can, but I always fall short.'

There can be no moratorium on brain research. It must go on, not only for practical reasons – it would be impossible to stop it throughout the world – nor for the gains that may be expected from it, but because it allows some of man's essential mysteries, such as the relationship between mind and body, to be studied scientifically for the first time.

Why can some critically ill persons apparently postpone the date of their own deaths until they have witnessed some event that is very important to them? Why do women who had been unable to conceive for years so often become pregnant shortly after they have adopted a child? Scientists can now investigate such phenomena, which may be linked to the production of various hormones in the brain. Even the pituitary, the body's 'master gland', must take orders from the hypothalamus. Various releasing hormones produced by the hypothalamus thus control growth, ovulation, the manufacture of sperm and one's reaction to stress. Once these hormones are better understood it will be possible to see how an idea or an emotion (e.g. faith, joy or fear) can change the brain's chemistry and thus affect the body's health.

As the life sciences increasingly focus on the brain, scientists are becoming more aware of the importance of purely psychological factors. Man's vulnerability to disease can some times be traced to specific brain mechanisms, and many intricate patterns of feedback are being uncovered.

At Rockefeller University, Dr Jay Weiss has shown how uncertainty, helplessness and fear lead to the development of stomach ulcers in rats that have been subjected to electric shocks while the same shocks do little or no damage to rats that are in a different frame of mind. His two sets of rats had identical electrodes wired in series on their tails, so that each received exactly the same painful electric shocks. But one partner in each set was kept ignorant of when the shocks were coming, while the other either received a signal of the impending shock or was given a chance to turn it off by pushing a lever. The ignorant and helpless rats lost weight, developed a high level of stress hormones in their blood, showed a low level of noradrenaline in their brains, and soon a great many of them had ulcers. The rats that knew what to expect remained fairly healthy. However, the rats that had a chance to turn off the shocks did even better: in addition to good health, they developed a high level of noradrenaline in their brains, which probably indicated a mood of euphoria. 'It is even conceivable that people need the challenge of successfully solving problems in order to maintain a happy mood,' suggested Dr Neal Miller, in whose lab those experiments took place.

If achievement brings health and euphoria, doubt about the value of one's efforts may bring illness, as further experimentation showed. When the rats found their tasks so unclear that they were never quite sure of being safe from shock, those that tried to cope but failed developed stomach ulcers much more frequently than their helpless partners. On the other hand, if the experimenter sounded a buzzer every time the rats performed correctly, thus confirming their good judgement as well as their safety, the rats became even healthier than before.

Philosophers used to ask, 'What is matter?' and reply jokingly, 'Never mind.' Psychologists asked, 'What is mind?' and replied, quite seriously, 'It doesn't matter.' Now the brain scientists are studying both mind and matter, together. They see that changes in a newborn rat's experiences can alter the size and chemistry of its brain, while various chemicals can affect its memory. Voluntary control of one's heart rate or blood pressure can produce changes in the electrical activity of one's brain, while electrical stimulation of the brain through electrodes can produce pain or pleasure. It is all leading to a new view of man, and for the first time, 'mental' therapies are beginning to make sense to hard-nosed scientists. At the same time, psychotherapists are looking at drug treatments with new respect.

As this new view develops, researchers are beginning to unravel our various states of consciousness – our sleep, our ecstasies, our anxieties and our reveries. They are exploring the differing qualities of our two cerebral hemispheres. They are studying the formation of our intentions and plans. Soon they will be able to study our emotions. Next they may begin to understand the greatest mystery of all: the act of creation, or how men produce the inventions and the new ideas that set them apart from all other living creatures.

Someday a scientist of genius will put all the pieces together and form a coherent picture of the brain. The technology is growing rapidly, some tentative links are already being formed between disparate findings and, around the year 2000, perhaps, the research findings will reach a critical mass. At that point, there will be an explosion of knowledge as startling as that of the first atomic bomb. Man's most private, most treasured possession – his brain – will lay exposed to public view. People will become powerful and vulnerable as never before. The issue of brain control will loom over them as ominously as that of atomic power hovers over us. What they make of it – whether their new power serves or destroys them – will depend to a large extent on what guidelines we set, and whether we keep a close watch on what the brain-changers are doing today.

Index

233

Index

Index